The Healing Spice Treasury

10 Indian Medicinal Spices Available in the Indian Kitchen

Dr.Khushboo

Copyright © <2025> <Dr.Khushboo>

Made with ♥ on the Notion Press Platform

www.notionpress.com

Table of Contents

Acknowledgements

Creating *The Healing Spice Treasury: 10 Indian Medicinal Spices Available in the Indian Kitchen* has been a deeply enriching journey, and it would not have been possible without the support, inspiration, and guidance of many incredible individuals and communities.

First and foremost, I want to express my gratitude to the traditional Indian healers, practitioners of Ayurveda, and culinary experts whose wisdom has inspired the contents of this book. Their age-old practices and knowledge form the backbone of this work, preserving the powerful legacy of using spices for health and healing. I am humbled by the depth of their insights and honoured to be able to share a small part of that wisdom with a broader audience.

To my husband and son thank you for teaching me that a kitchen is more than a place for cooking; it is a sanctuary of wellness and love. From childhood memories of fragrant spices wafting through our home to the practical lessons of spice blending and remedy-making, your influence runs deeply through every page of this book.

Special thanks go to my mother and my father who have guided my understanding of traditional Indian medicinal spices and holistic healing. Your encouragement and expertise have been invaluable, and I am grateful for the guidance, feedback, and time you generously offered throughout this project.

Lastly, I would like to acknowledge the readers who are passionate about natural health and strive to find healing and nourishment in everyday ingredients. This book is for you—a celebration of the beauty, wisdom, and power hidden in the spice jars on our shelves. Thank you for joining me on this journey into the heart of Indian kitchen remedies. I hope this book brings you as much joy, healing, and discovery as it has brought me in writing it.

With gratitude and warmth,

[Dr.Khushboo]

Introduction

Welcome to the vibrant, aromatic world of Indian spices! Imagine opening a simple kitchen cabinet and discovering a treasure trove of natural remedies ready to soothe, heal, and energize you. In India, spices are more than just culinary add-ons; they're trusted companions for health, wellness, and healing. From helping a scratchy throat to easing a bad case of indigestion, Indian spices bring centuries of medicinal wisdom to the table, all from ingredients you can easily find at home. It's like having a personal pharmacy in your pantry, one that smells delightful, tastes incredible and doesn't come with a long list of side effects.

India's spice history dates back thousands of years, with roots stretching into the origins of Ayurveda—one of the world's oldest holistic healing systems. For thousands of years, spices have played a role in adding flavour and aroma to meals and enhancing vitality, treating ailments, and fortifying the immune system. These little seeds, leaves, and roots carry potent medicinal properties, often recognised today by modern science for the benefits ancient cultures already understood. This book dives into ten powerhouse spices that have stood the test of time, highlighting their uses, healing properties, and simple ways to incorporate them into your daily routine.

The Healing Power of Spices

Indian medicinal spices are more than remedies—they are an integral part of the cultural and culinary landscape. They appear in the morning cup of *chai*, in the midday curry, and even in the simple act of chewing on fennel seeds after meals. The healing potential of these spices is vast, and they are often the first line of treatment for minor ailments. From a sore throat to digestive discomfort, Indian families rely on the kitchen for instant relief before turning to other treatments. This makes the kitchen a natural pharmacy, where health and flavour go hand in hand.

Furthermore, these spices support preventive care, not just reactive treatment. By incorporating them into everyday meals, they offer consistent health benefits, helping to build immunity, manage blood sugar levels, and promote cardiovascular health, among other benefits. For example, cinnamon and fenugreek have been shown to help regulate blood sugar levels, making them beneficial for people with or at risk of diabetes. Cloves and black pepper, on the other hand, are known for their antimicrobial properties, which aid in combating infections and boosting the body's natural defenses.

Here's a taste of what awaits you inside each chapter:

Turmeric – The Golden Healer

Ever wondered why your curry has a warm, golden hue? Meet turmeric, the "Golden Healer," packed with curcumin, an antioxidant and anti-inflammatory powerhouse. Known for its anti-inflammatory and antibacterial properties, turmeric is a go-to for everything from sprains to colds. Mixed in warm milk or added to food, this spice is India's answer to nature's antibiotic and a gentle healer for body and mind.

Ginger – Nature's Digestive Aid

Ginger is a knobby root that looks ordinary on the outside but holds a world of health benefits inside. From calming an upset stomach to easing arthritis pain, ginger's versatility is legendary. Whether you use it fresh, dried, or powdered, this spice works wonders as a digestive aid, helping with everything from nausea to bloating. Add it to tea, soup, or a refreshing juice, and let it work its soothing magic on your digestive system.

Cumin – The Digestion Enhancer

If you've ever enjoyed the earthy, nutty taste of cumin, you're already familiar with its flavor-boosting prowess. But did you know cumin is also a fantastic digestion enhancer? Known for stimulating enzyme production, cumin can help tackle indigestion, bloating, and more. A pinch of roasted cumin in your buttermilk or sprinkled over vegetables can give your gut the gentle help it needs to feel at ease.

Coriander – The Cooling Companion

Coriander seeds are like little cooling warriors, calming the body and promoting digestive health. Known for their diuretic and detoxifying properties, coriander seeds are excellent for balancing pitta (the fire element) in Ayurvedic traditions. Their subtle citrusy flavor is perfect in soups, stews, or teas, adding a gentle touch of flavor while helping the body stay balanced and refreshed.

Fenugreek – The Blood Sugar Balancer

Fenugreek seeds may be small, but their impact on health is mighty. Known for balancing blood sugar levels, fenugreek also supports lactation in new mothers and helps in digestion. These slightly bitter seeds add depth to curries and can be consumed as a tea for a natural health boost, especially for those managing diabetes or looking to boost their metabolism.

Cinnamon – The Circulation Stimulator

Cinnamon is the warm, sweet spice that makes everything from tea to dessert feel cozy. But it's more than just a flavor enhancer; cinnamon is a circulation booster and can even help regulate blood sugar. Known for its antioxidant, anti-inflammatory, and antimicrobial properties, a pinch of cinnamon can be added to your morning tea or oatmeal to give your metabolism and immunity a gentle boost.

Cloves – The Powerful Pain Reliever

These tiny buds pack a punch! Cloves are celebrated for their pain-relieving and antiseptic properties, especially in oral health. From soothing a toothache to reducing inflammation, cloves have been trusted for ages to fight off bacteria and provide relief. Pop a clove into your tea or chew one gently to enjoy its aromatic warmth and natural pain-relief properties.

Black Pepper – The Immunity Booster

Black pepper, or "the King of Spices," is well-known for adding a spicy kick to food, but did you know it's also a powerful immune booster? Rich in piperine, black pepper enhances the absorption of other nutrients (like curcumin in turmeric), fights off cold and cough symptoms, and helps digestion. A pinch in your food can give a natural immunity boost and add depth of flavor to any dish.

Cardamom – The Queen of Calm

Known as the "Queen of Spices," cardamom is both soothing and refreshing. Its delicate, sweet aroma is a staple in chai tea, but this spice is also an effective digestive aid and breath freshener. Cardamom's ability to cool the digestive tract makes it perfect for balancing heat, promoting calmness, and reducing stress. Add it to your tea or chew a pod for a fresh, relaxing lift.

Fennel – The Gentle Detoxifier

Fennel is like a breath of fresh air for your digestive system. Known for its sweet licorice taste, fennel is excellent for detoxifying the body, reducing bloating, and improving digestion. After a heavy meal, chewing on fennel seeds or brewing a fennel tea can help you feel light and refreshed. Its mild properties make it safe for daily use and beneficial for maintaining digestive health.

Why You'll Love These Spices

You don't need a special pantry or a degree in botany to benefit from these spices—they're right there in your kitchen, ready to add flavour and wellness to your life. Each chapter of this book highlights one powerful spice, explaining its benefits, unique properties, and fun ways to enjoy it. Whether you're battling seasonal sniffles, feeling a little bloated, or just need a natural pick-me-up, these spices have you covered.

How to Use This Book

This book is not just a guide; it's an invitation to get creative and curious. Each chapter breaks down the health benefits of one spice, along with simple recipes and tips on how to incorporate it into your daily routine. You don't have to be a chef or a health guru—just a little adventurous in the kitchen. So grab your spice jars, boil some water for tea, and dive in!

Final Thoughts

As you turn the pages, you'll learn about the science, traditions, and healing powers of these 10 Indian medicinal spices that can turn any kitchen into a wellness sanctuary. From enhancing immunity to boosting mood and digestion, each of these spices is like a little helper, working to keep you feeling great. By the end of this journey, you'll have a renewed appreciation for the everyday spices in your kitchen and feel empowered to use them in ways that elevate your health and well-being.

With their humble yet powerful presence, these spices remind us that sometimes, the best medicine comes from nature— simple, accessible, and full of life-giving energy. Here's to finding health, balance, and flavour in the magic of Indian spices!

Let's get started! ☺

1 Chapter 1: Turmeric – The Golden Healer

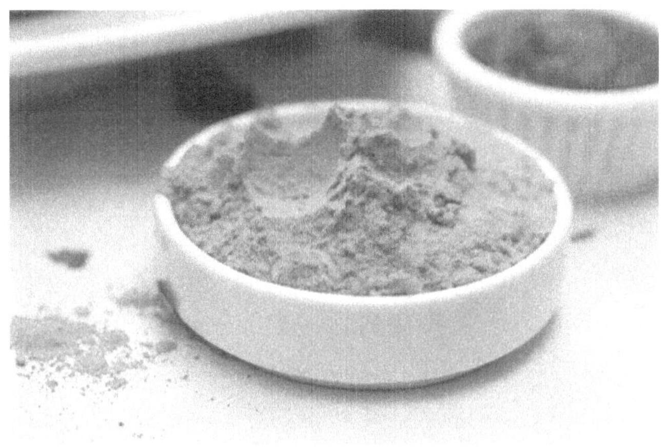

Introduction

Turmeric, or *Haldi* in Hindi, is often called the "golden spice" of India, celebrated not only for its vibrant yellow hue but also for its powerful healing properties. This ancient spice, derived from the root of the *Curcuma longa* plant, has been used for thousands of years in Indian cooking, traditional medicine, and religious rituals. Turmeric's unique medicinal importance lies primarily in its active compound, curcumin, which is responsible for its bright colour and numerous health benefits. Revered in Ayurveda and increasingly validated by modern science, turmeric is a natural remedy with anti-inflammatory, antioxidant, and antimicrobial properties, making it a staple in Indian kitchens and healing practices.

Medicinal Importance of Turmeric

Turmeric has gained the title of "Golden Healer" due to its extensive medicinal benefits. Here's an in-depth look at its therapeutic properties and the ways in which it supports various aspects of health.

1. Anti-Inflammatory Properties

Curcumin, the active component of turmeric, is renowned for its strong anti-inflammatory effects, which are comparable to some over-the-counter anti-inflammatory drugs but without harmful side effects. Inflammation is a natural bodily response, but chronic inflammation has been linked to many diseases, including arthritis, heart disease, and cancer. Turmeric helps to reduce inflammation in the body, alleviating symptoms of conditions like arthritis, and promoting joint health.

- **Home Remedy for Arthritis**: Mix one teaspoon of turmeric powder with warm milk or water and a pinch of black pepper (which enhances curcumin absorption) to help relieve joint pain and stiffness.

2. Powerful Antioxidant

Turmeric is a potent antioxidant, which helps neutralize free radicals in the body. Free radicals can damage cells and lead to premature ageing and diseases like cancer, Alzheimer's, and cardiovascular disorders. Curcumin not only combats free radicals directly but also boosts the body's own antioxidant defences, making it highly effective in promoting cellular health and reducing the oxidative stress that leads to chronic diseases.

- **Anti-Aging Drink**: Turmeric tea, or "Golden Milk," made with turmeric, black pepper, and a pinch of cinnamon in milk, can be enjoyed daily to reduce oxidative stress and improve overall health.

3. Boosts Immunity

In Ayurveda, turmeric is considered a natural immunity booster, often used as a preventative measure to keep infections at bay. Its antimicrobial, antiviral, and antibacterial properties make it an excellent remedy for colds, coughs, and respiratory issues. Additionally, the immune-boosting effects of turmeric may help reduce the frequency and severity of common illnesses.

- **Immunity-Boosting Drink**: A mixture of turmeric, ginger, and honey in warm water can be taken daily to strengthen immunity, especially during cold and flu season.

4. Supports Digestive Health

Turmeric aids in digestion by stimulating bile production, which helps break down fats. It also reduces symptoms of bloating and gas, making it an effective remedy for those with digestive issues. Moreover, turmeric's anti-inflammatory properties can help alleviate symptoms of inflammatory bowel disease (IBD) and irritable bowel syndrome (IBS).

- **Digestive Aid**: Adding a pinch of turmeric to meals, or drinking warm water with turmeric before meals, can improve digestion and reduce bloating.

5. Promotes Heart Health

Curcumin supports heart health by improving the function of the endothelium, which is the lining of blood vessels. Endothelial dysfunction is a major driver of heart disease, as it affects blood pressure and blood clotting. By enhancing endothelial function and reducing inflammation and oxidation, turmeric can lower the risk of heart disease. Curcumin also helps reduce cholesterol levels, promoting a healthier cardiovascular system.

- **Heart Health Mix**: Combine turmeric with honey and a pinch of black pepper to create a daily spoonful that can be added to smoothies or warm water for heart support.

6. May Help Prevent and Treat Cancer

Research suggests that curcumin has the potential to influence cancer development, growth, and spread at the molecular level. Curcumin has been shown to reduce the growth of cancerous cells and may even prevent the formation of tumours. While turmeric alone is not a cure, it may complement traditional cancer treatments by reducing tumour growth and enhancing the effectiveness of chemotherapy.

- **Cancer-Prevention Supplement**: Though not a replacement for medical treatment, turmeric supplements can be considered under the guidance of a healthcare professional to support cancer therapy.

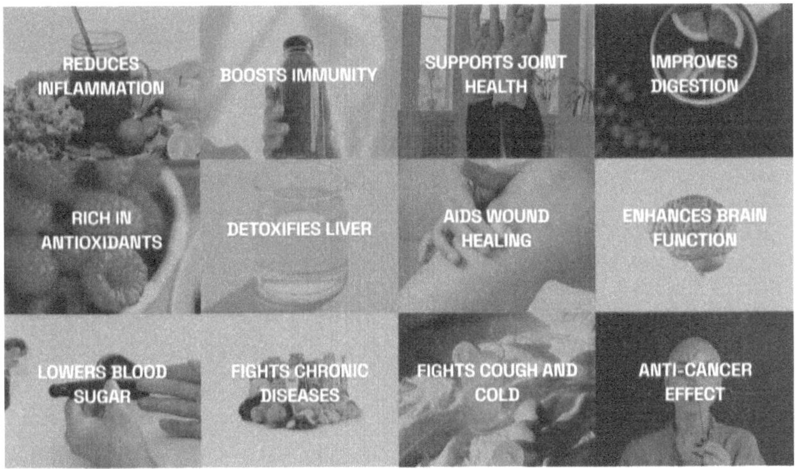

7. Supports Brain Health and Reduces Risk of Neurodegenerative Diseases

Curcumin has shown promise in supporting brain health by increasing levels of brain-derived neurotrophic factor (BDNF), a protein that promotes the growth and survival of neurons. Low levels of BDNF are associated with neurodegenerative diseases like Alzheimer's and depression. By boosting BDNF levels, turmeric may help delay or reverse brain degeneration. Additionally, its antioxidant properties protect the brain from oxidative damage, another factor in neurodegeneration.

- **Brain Health Remedy**: A daily dose of turmeric in tea or milk may help improve cognitive function and reduce the risk of Alzheimer's when consumed regularly.

8. Promotes Skin Health

Turmeric has been used in traditional skincare routines for its anti-inflammatory, antimicrobial, and antioxidant benefits. It helps treat acne, reduces blemishes, and brightens the skin tone. Turmeric's ability to reduce inflammation and bacteria on the skin makes it a popular ingredient in masks and other skincare preparations. When applied topically, turmeric can soothe skin conditions like eczema, psoriasis, and dermatitis.

- **Skin Glow Mask**: Make a paste with turmeric, honey, and yogurt and apply it to the face. Leave it on for 10-15 minutes, then rinse off to enjoy a brighter complexion and reduced inflammation.

Turmeric in Everyday Life

Turmeric is versatile and can be easily added to daily meals, from curries to rice dishes, soups, and teas. Its distinct colour and flavour make it an integral part of Indian cuisine, and with the additional health benefits, it's a spice worth including in every diet. Here are a few practical ways to incorporate turmeric into your routine:

- **Golden Milk**: A warm blend of milk (or plant milk), turmeric, black pepper, and a pinch of cinnamon, sweetened with honey, is a traditional nighttime drink that supports sleep, digestion, and immunity.

- **Daily Cooking**: Adding turmeric to curries, soups, and rice dishes enhances flavour and delivers daily benefits without any extra effort.

- **Turmeric Paste**: A homemade turmeric paste made with turmeric, black pepper, and coconut oil can be stored and added to dishes or warm beverages as needed.

21

Ayurvedic Context of Turmeric

In Ayurveda, turmeric (*Curcuma longa*), known as *Haridra* in Sanskrit, is revered as one of the most potent and versatile medicinal spices. Its vibrant golden color and unique properties have earned it the title of the "Golden Healer." Turmeric is considered a sacred plant in Ayurvedic tradition, symbolizing purity, prosperity, and protection. Its use in medicine, rituals, and cuisine dates back over 5,000 years, and it continues to be a cornerstone of holistic health practices.

Dosha Balancing Properties

According to Ayurveda, turmeric possesses a bitter (*tikta*) and pungent (*katu*) taste, with a heating (*ushna*) effect on the body. It primarily balances the *Kapha* and *Vata* doshas while slightly aggravating *Pitta* when consumed in excess. Turmeric's heating quality helps to stimulate digestion, clear mucus, and improve circulation, making it beneficial for individuals with sluggish metabolism or cold-related imbalances.

Turmeric as a Natural Detoxifier

Turmeric is highly valued for its detoxifying and cleansing properties. It is believed to purify the blood (*rakta shodhana*), enhance liver function, and eliminate toxins (*ama*) from the body. This detoxifying action supports healthy skin, boosts immunity, and promotes overall vitality. Turmeric is often incorporated into Ayurvedic cleanses and seasonal detox routines to rejuvenate the body and mind.

Anti-Inflammatory and Healing Properties

In Ayurveda, inflammation (*shotha*) is viewed as a root cause of many diseases. Turmeric's active compound, curcumin, is renowned for its potent anti-inflammatory properties. It is used to treat conditions such as arthritis, joint pain, and muscle stiffness. Ayurvedic practitioners often recommend turmeric in combination with warm milk or ghee to enhance its absorption and efficacy in reducing inflammation.

Digestive and Immune Support

Turmeric is considered a powerful digestive aid (*dipana*) in Ayurveda. It stimulates the secretion of digestive enzymes, enhances appetite, and alleviates bloating and gas. Additionally, its antimicrobial and immune-boosting properties protect the body from infections and respiratory ailments. Turmeric is a common remedy for colds, coughs, and sore throats, often combined with honey or black pepper for enhanced effectiveness.

Spiritual and Ritual Significance

Beyond its medicinal uses, turmeric holds a special place in Ayurvedic rituals and spiritual practices. It is applied to the forehead as a symbol of the third eye, representing spiritual awakening and protection from negative energies. Turmeric paste is also used in ceremonies and weddings to purify and bless individuals.

In essence, turmeric embodies the holistic philosophy of Ayurveda, offering physical, mental, and spiritual benefits. Its versatility and efficacy make it a timeless remedy for health and well-being.

Precautions

While turmeric is generally safe, high doses of curcumin supplements may cause digestive upset and interact with medications, especially blood thinners. It's also advisable to consult a healthcare provider before using turmeric supplements, especially for those with gallbladder issues or bleeding disorders.

Conclusion

Turmeric's potent healing powers and versatility make it a true "Golden Healer." By adding this ancient spice into your daily routine, you can harness its numerous health benefits while enjoying its vibrant flavour. Whether as a remedy for inflammation, an immune booster, or support for skin and brain health, turmeric continues to be a beloved and essential spice for wellness, bridging the gap between traditional wisdom and modern science.

<u>RECIPES</u>

Here are 10 medicinal recipes featuring turmeric, a versatile spice known for its powerful anti-inflammatory, antioxidant, and immune-boosting properties. These recipes are designed to help with various health concerns and easily incorporate into daily life.

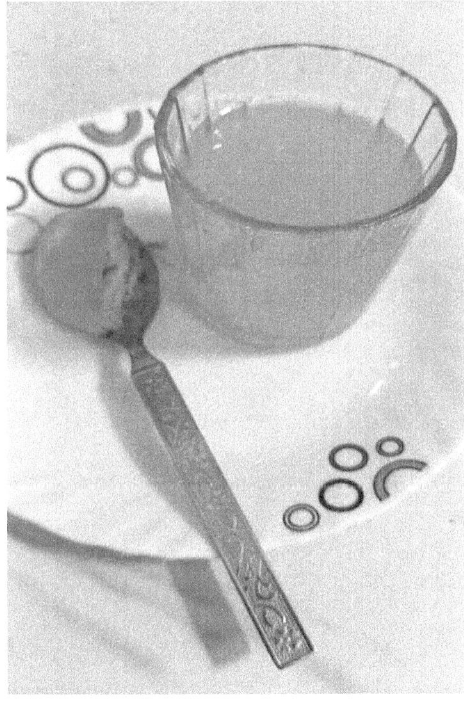

1. Turmeric Tea

Turmeric Tea for Detoxification and Digestion

This tea can help with detox, boost digestion, and is great for reducing bloating.

Ingredients:

- 1/2 teaspoon turmeric powder (or a small piece of fresh turmeric root, grated)

- 1 cup hot water

- A squeeze of lemon juice

- Honey or ginger (optional, for added benefits)

Instructions:

1. Mix turmeric powder with hot water, stirring well.

2. Add lemon juice, honey, or ginger if desired.

3. Drink warm, especially after meals, to aid digestion and support liver health.

2. Turmeric Golden Milk (Haldi Doodh)

A traditional remedy for better immunity and restful sleep.
Ingredients:

- 1 cup milk (dairy or plant-based)
- 1/2 teaspoon turmeric powder
- A pinch of black pepper
- 1/4 teaspoon cinnamon (optional)
- 1 teaspoon honey or jaggery

Instructions:

1. Heat milk, add turmeric, black pepper, and cinnamon.

2. Simmer for 5 minutes, then sweeten with honey or jaggery.

Benefits: Reduces inflammation, soothes colds, and aids sleep.

3. Turmeric and Ginger Tea

A detox tea to fight colds and support digestion.
Ingredients:

- 1 cup water

- 1/2 teaspoon turmeric powder or grated fresh turmeric

- 1-inch ginger (grated)

- Lemon juice and honey (optional)

Instructions:

1. Boil water, add turmeric and ginger, and simmer for 10 minutes.

2. Strain, add lemon juice or honey for taste.

Benefits: Boosts immunity, eases nausea, and soothes sore throats.

4. Turmeric Lemon Water

A refreshing detox drink for energy and cleansing.
Ingredients:

- 1 cup warm water

- 1/2 teaspoon turmeric powder

- Juice of 1/2 lemon

- A pinch of black pepper

Instructions:

1. Mix all ingredients into warm water and drink on an empty stomach.

Benefits: Promotes digestion, detoxifies, and improves skin health.

5. Turmeric Face Mask

A topical remedy for glowing skin.
Ingredients:

- 1 teaspoon turmeric powder

- 2 tablespoons yogurt or milk

- 1 teaspoon honey

Instructions:

1. Mix into a paste and apply to the face.

2. Leave for 10–15 minutes, then rinse off.

Benefits: Reduces acne, brightens skin, and soothes inflammation.

6. Turmeric Rice for Joint Health

A simple dish packed with anti-inflammatory benefits.
Ingredients:

- 1 cup cooked rice

- 1/2 teaspoon turmeric powder

- A pinch of black pepper

- 1 teaspoon ghee or olive oil

Instructions:

1. Mix turmeric and black pepper into warm rice.

2. Add ghee or olive oil and serve warm.

Benefits: Reduces joint pain and supports digestion.

7. Turmeric and Garlic Soup

A healing soup to fight colds and flu.
Ingredients:

- 2 cups vegetable or chicken broth

- 1 teaspoon turmeric powder

- 2 garlic cloves (crushed)

- 1 cup coconut milk

Instructions:

1. Simmer broth, turmeric, and garlic for 10 minutes.

2. Add coconut milk and serve warm.

Benefits: Boosts immunity, soothes inflammation, and fights infections.

8. Turmeric Smoothie

A tasty drink for energy and inflammation relief.
Ingredients:

- 1 cup almond or coconut milk

- 1/2 teaspoon turmeric powder

- 1 banana

- 1/4 teaspoon ginger powder

- 1 teaspoon honey

Instructions:

1. Blend all ingredients until smooth and enjoy chilled.

Benefits: Boosts energy, fights inflammation, and improves digestion.

9. Turmeric Oil for Topical Use

A healing oil for wounds and joint pain.
Ingredients:

- 1/4 cup coconut or olive oil

- 1 tablespoon turmeric powder

Instructions:

1. Mix turmeric into the oil and gently warm it.

2. Apply to wounds or sore joints.

Benefits: Speeds healing, reduces inflammation, and soothes pain.

10. Turmeric Pickle (Haldi Achaar)

A tangy probiotic-rich health booster.
Ingredients:

- 1 cup fresh turmeric root (sliced)

- Juice of 2 lemons

- 1 teaspoon mustard seeds

- Salt to taste

Instructions:

1. Mix all ingredients and let marinate for 1–2 days.

2. Store in the refrigerator and enjoy with meals.

Benefits: Improves digestion, supports gut health, and boosts immunity.

Common Myths and Misconceptions About Turmeric

Turmeric is celebrated globally for its medicinal properties but has also become the subject of myths and misconceptions. Let's separate fact from fiction to understand its true potential.

1. Turmeric Can Cure All Diseases

Myth: Turmeric is a magical cure-all for every ailment, from the common cold to cancer.

Reality: While turmeric, particularly its active compound curcumin, has proven health benefits, it is not a standalone cure for serious conditions like cancer or chronic diseases. It can support treatment and improve health when combined with a balanced diet and lifestyle but should not replace medical interventions.

2. More Turmeric Means Better Results

Myth: The more turmeric you consume, the greater the health benefits.

Reality: Excessive turmeric consumption can cause side effects like nausea, diarrhoea, or dizziness. Moderation is key, and a daily intake of 500–2000 mg of curcumin (found in turmeric) is generally considered safe for most people.

3. Turmeric Works Instantly

Myth: Drinking turmeric tea or using a turmeric face mask will provide immediate results.

Reality: The benefits of turmeric, whether for health or skincare, are cumulative and require consistent use over time. Instant relief or results are unlikely.

4. Turmeric Has No Side Effects

Myth: Turmeric is 100% safe and has no side effects.

Reality: While turmeric is generally safe, excessive use or sensitivity can cause allergic reactions, stomach upset, or interaction with medications like blood thinners. Consult a doctor if you have pre-existing conditions.

5. Turmeric Is Only Beneficial When Eaten

Myth: The only way to benefit from turmeric is by consuming it.

Reality: Turmeric can also be applied topically to treat skin conditions, used as an antiseptic for wounds, or inhaled as part of steam therapy for colds. Its versatility goes beyond ingestion.

6. Turmeric and Curcumin Are the Same

Myth: Turmeric and curcumin are interchangeable terms.

Reality: Curcumin is one of the active compounds in turmeric that gives it its bright yellow color and many of its medicinal properties. However, turmeric also contains other compounds that contribute to its overall benefits.

7. Turmeric Works Without Any Additives

Myth: Turmeric doesn't need anything else to be effective.

Reality: Turmeric's active compound, curcumin, is poorly absorbed by the body on its own. Combining it with black pepper (containing piperine) or healthy fats significantly enhances its bioavailability and effectiveness.

8. Cooking Turmeric Destroys Its Benefits

Myth: Heating turmeric during cooking eliminates its medicinal properties.

Reality: Moderate heat does not destroy turmeric's benefits and may even enhance curcumin's bioavailability. Overheating for prolonged periods might reduce its potency, so use it wisely in cooking.

9. Only Raw Turmeric Is Effective

Myth: Fresh turmeric root is superior to powdered turmeric.

Reality: Both forms are beneficial, but the choice depends on how you use them. Fresh turmeric may have a stronger flavor and slightly more nutrients, while powdered turmeric is convenient and still highly effective.

10. Turmeric Is a New Superfood Trend

Myth: Turmeric has only recently gained popularity as a superfood.

Reality: Turmeric has been used for over 4,000 years in Indian Ayurvedic and traditional medicine systems. Its recent popularity in the West as a "superfood" is a rediscovery of this ancient ingredient.

By dispelling these myths, we can fully appreciate turmeric for what it truly is: a powerful, versatile spice with immense potential for promoting health and well-being—when used correctl

Chapter 2: Ginger – Nature's Digestive Aid

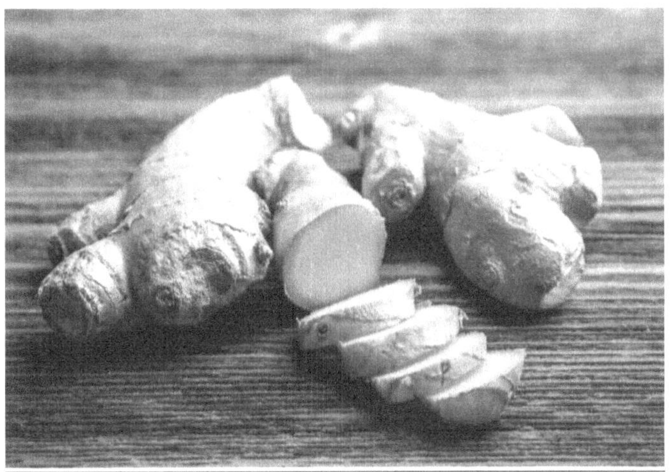

Introduction

Ginger, known as *Adrak* in Hindi, is a warming, aromatic root that has been used for thousands of years as both a culinary ingredient and a medicinal powerhouse. Derived from the *Zingiber officinale* plant, ginger's popularity in traditional medicine spans across Ayurveda, Chinese medicine, and other holistic systems. Often referred to as "Nature's Digestive Aid," ginger is prized for its ability to promote digestion, reduce nausea, and soothe inflammation. Its unique flavor and myriad health benefits make it a staple in kitchens worldwide, especially in Indian households, where it's commonly added to tea, curries, and remedies for various ailments.

This chapter delves into the medicinal properties of ginger, exploring its benefits for digestive health, immunity, pain relief, and more. With its versatility and effectiveness, ginger remains a cornerstone of natural healing practices, continuing to earn its place as one of the most valuable spices in the kitchen.

Medicinal Importance of Ginger

Ginger's rich bioactive compounds, including gingerol, shogaol, and zingerone, are responsible for its many health-promoting effects. Here's a closer look at the medicinal benefits of ginger and how it can be used to support various aspects of health.

1. Digestive Health

Ginger is widely known for its ability to support digestion. Its natural compounds stimulate the production of digestive enzymes, which help break down food more efficiently. Ginger is also effective in reducing gas, bloating, and discomfort associated with indigestion. By stimulating gastric emptying and promoting a smooth digestive process, ginger can be a reliable remedy for various digestive disorders.

- **Home Remedy for Indigestion**: Sipping on ginger tea made by boiling fresh ginger in water can ease indigestion and soothe the stomach. Consuming a small piece of raw ginger with salt before meals is also a traditional way to stimulate digestion.

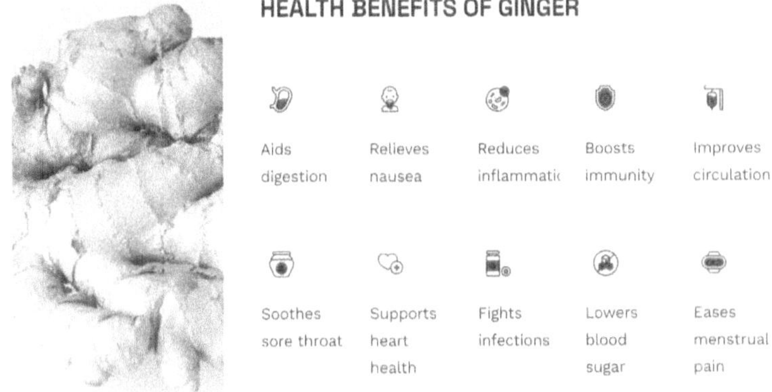

2. Anti-nausea and Anti-Vomiting

One of ginger's most well-known uses is for alleviating nausea. Ginger has shown significant efficacy in reducing nausea and vomiting, particularly in cases of motion sickness, morning sickness during pregnancy, and post-operative nausea. Its anti-nausea effects make it a natural alternative to over-the-counter medications, especially for those seeking gentle relief.

- **Nausea Relief**: Chewing on a small piece of ginger, or drinking ginger tea, can help relieve nausea. For pregnancy-related morning sickness, ginger capsules or tea provide a safe and effective solution.

3. Anti-Inflammatory Properties

Ginger's potent anti-inflammatory properties make it an effective remedy for various inflammatory conditions. The active compounds in ginger, especially gingerol, have been shown to reduce inflammation and inhibit pain-causing compounds. This makes ginger beneficial for managing conditions like arthritis, muscle soreness, and joint pain.

- **Pain Relief for Arthritis**: Regularly consuming ginger tea or adding ginger powder to meals can help reduce arthritis pain and stiffness. For topical relief, a warm ginger poultice can be applied to sore joints to ease inflammation.

4. Supports Immunity

In Ayurveda, ginger is often referred to as a "heating" herb, which means it has the power to increase circulation, boost metabolism, and fight infections. Ginger's antimicrobial and antiviral properties help support the immune system and fend off colds, coughs, and infections. By encouraging sweating, ginger can also help the body detoxify and recover more quickly from illnesses.

- **Cold and Flu Remedy**: A soothing ginger, honey, and lemon tea is a popular remedy to help reduce cold and flu symptoms. Ginger tea with honey can also relieve sore throats and coughs, making it ideal during colder months.

5. Cardiovascular Health

Ginger contributes to heart health by reducing inflammation, improving circulation, and helping to regulate cholesterol levels. Studies have shown that ginger can lower blood pressure and reduce blood clotting, both of which help decrease the risk of heart disease. By improving circulation, ginger also promotes better oxygenation and nutrient flow throughout the body.

- **Heart-Healthy Ginger Tea**: Consuming ginger tea or adding ginger to daily meals can help support cardiovascular health. Adding a pinch of cinnamon enhances its heart-healthy effects.

6. Blood Sugar Regulation

Research has shown that ginger may help manage blood sugar levels by improving insulin sensitivity and lowering fasting blood sugar levels. This is particularly beneficial for individuals with diabetes or those at risk of developing type 2 diabetes. Regular consumption of ginger can help stabilize blood sugar levels, which may improve energy and reduce the risk of diabetic complications.

- **Blood Sugar Balancer**: Drinking ginger tea or adding ginger powder to meals, especially in combination with cinnamon, can help regulate blood sugar levels. A small piece of fresh ginger before meals may also aid in blood sugar control.

7. Pain Relief and Muscle Soreness

Ginger's anti-inflammatory and analgesic properties make it an effective natural remedy for muscle pain and soreness, particularly after exercise. Studies have shown that consuming ginger daily can help reduce muscle pain and accelerate recovery time after physical activity. Its warming nature can also help soothe sore muscles and promote relaxation.

- **Exercise Recovery Drink**: A post-workout drink made with ginger, lemon, and a touch of honey can help reduce muscle soreness and speed up recovery.

8. Promotes Respiratory Health

Ginger is a natural expectorant, which means it can help loosen mucus and phlegm, making it easier to expel from the respiratory system. This is particularly beneficial for those with respiratory conditions like asthma, bronchitis, or chronic coughs. Ginger's warming effects also soothe sore throats and reduce chest congestion, making it ideal for respiratory relief.

- **Respiratory Relief**: Ginger tea with honey and a dash of black pepper can be a natural remedy for congestion and respiratory discomfort. Consuming this mixture regularly can help clear up congestion and support respiratory health.

9. Menstrual Pain Relief

For centuries, ginger has been used as a natural remedy for menstrual pain and cramps. The anti-inflammatory compounds in ginger help reduce pain and discomfort by relaxing the muscles and easing cramps. Some studies suggest that ginger can be as effective as over-the-counter pain relievers for menstrual pain.

- **Menstrual Cramp Tea**: A cup of warm ginger tea or a small piece of raw ginger taken at the onset of menstrual pain can provide relief. Adding a pinch of turmeric can enhance the anti-inflammatory effects.

10. Anti-Cancer Potential

Research indicates that ginger may play a role in inhibiting the growth of cancer cells and reducing the risk of certain cancers, including colon and ovarian cancer. The antioxidant and anti-inflammatory properties of ginger help protect cells from damage, which can reduce cancer risk. While ginger is not a cure for cancer, it is increasingly recognized as a supportive measure in a healthy lifestyle.

- **Cancer Prevention Supplement**: Including ginger in the diet or as a tea may help reduce cancer risk. However, it's always best to consult a healthcare provider before using ginger supplements for specific health conditions.

Incorporating Ginger into Daily Life

Ginger is a versatile spice that can be easily incorporated into daily meals and beverages. From ginger tea to adding fresh ginger to soups, stir-fries, and curries, there are countless ways to enjoy its health benefits. Here are a few practical tips:

- **Ginger Tea**: Boil a few slices of fresh ginger in water for 10-15 minutes. Add honey and lemon for a soothing, health-boosting drink.

- **Cooking**: Grate fresh ginger into curries, soups, or marinades to add a burst of flavor and promote digestive health.

- **Ginger and Honey Paste**: A mix of ginger juice and honey can be taken daily to support immunity and relieve sore throats.

Ayurvedic Context of Ginger

In Ayurveda, ginger (*Zingiber officinale*), known as *Adraka* (fresh ginger) and *Shunthi* (dried ginger) in Sanskrit, is celebrated as the "Universal Medicine" (*Vishwabhesaj*). Its widespread use in Ayurvedic practices, both as a culinary spice and a therapeutic herb, highlights its versatility and potency in promoting health and well-being. Ginger is considered a cornerstone of Ayurvedic medicine, offering a range of benefits for the body, mind, and spirit.

Dosha Balancing Properties

Ginger is a tri-doshic herb, meaning it can balance all three doshas—*Vata*, *Pitta*, and *Kapha*—though it is most effective in pacifying *Vata* and *Kapha*. Its pungent (*katu*) taste, heating (*ushna*) energy, and light (*laghu*) qualities help to stimulate the digestive fire (*Agni*), making it an essential remedy for cold, stagnant, or sluggish conditions. However, excessive consumption may aggravate *Pitta* due to its heat-inducing properties.

Digestive and Metabolic Enhancer

Ginger is renowned in Ayurveda as a powerful digestive aid (*dipana*) and carminative (*anulomana*). It enhances appetite, stimulates the secretion of digestive enzymes, and promotes the efficient breakdown of food. It is particularly effective in alleviating symptoms of indigestion, bloating, gas, and nausea. Fresh ginger juice mixed with a pinch of rock salt and lime is a common Ayurvedic remedy to ignite the digestive fire and relieve gastrointestinal discomfort.

Anti-Inflammatory and Pain Relief

In Ayurveda, inflammation (*shotha*) is seen as a root cause of many chronic diseases. Ginger's anti-inflammatory properties are highly valued for reducing pain and swelling associated with conditions such as arthritis, muscle aches, and joint stiffness. Dried ginger powder, when combined with honey and warm water, is often prescribed to alleviate chronic inflammation and enhance joint flexibility.

Immune Booster and Respiratory Support

Ginger is considered a natural immune booster (*Rasayana*) due to its antimicrobial and antiviral properties. It helps to ward off common colds, flu, and respiratory infections by clearing mucus, relieving congestion, and soothing a sore throat. A traditional Ayurvedic remedy for respiratory health involves brewing fresh ginger tea with tulsi (holy basil) and honey to strengthen the immune system and support lung function.

Circulatory and Detoxifying Agent

Ginger is known to enhance blood circulation and support cardiovascular health. Its ability to stimulate circulation makes it beneficial for individuals with cold hands and feet or poor blood flow. Additionally, its detoxifying properties help to eliminate toxins (*ama*) from the body, promoting overall vitality and energy.

In Ayurveda, ginger is more than just a spice—it is a holistic healer that harmonizes the body's internal systems, offering warmth, energy, and balance to the body and mind.

Precautions

While ginger is generally safe, excessive consumption may cause mild digestive upset. Those on blood-thinning medications or with gallbladder issues should consult a healthcare provider before using ginger supplements or consuming large amounts, as ginger may interfere with blood clotting.

Conclusion

With its long history as a digestive aid and overall health booster, ginger lives up to its title as "Nature's Digestive Aid." Its anti-inflammatory, antimicrobial, and antioxidant properties make it an essential part of natural healing practices. Whether used to soothe an upset stomach, alleviate nausea, or boost immunity, ginger remains a valuable spice with a wealth of medicinal benefits. Including ginger in your daily routine can transform your kitchen into a center of wellness, offering nature's own remedy for a range of ailments.

<u>RECIPES</u>

1. Ginger Tea for Digestion and Nausea Relief

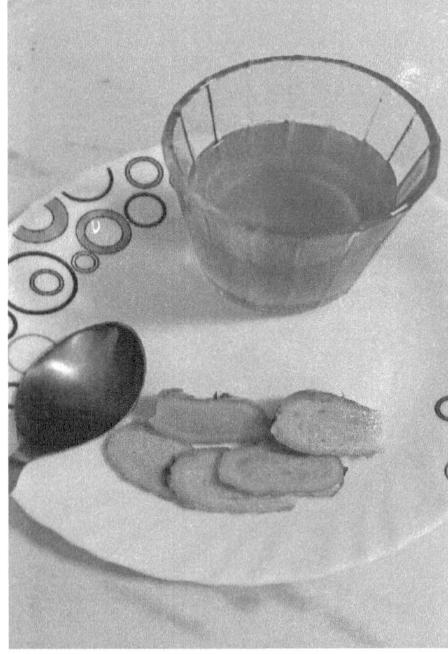

Ginger tea helps relieve nausea, indigestion, bloating and menstrual pain.

Ingredients:

- 1-2 inches of fresh ginger root, sliced (or 1 teaspoon ginger powder)

- 2 cups water

- Honey or lemon (optional, for added flavor)

Instructions:

1. Boil the water and add ginger slices.

2. Simmer for 10-15 minutes, then strain into a cup.

3. Add honey or lemon if desired, and drink warm.

2. Ginger and Honey Cough Syrup

This homemade syrup is effective for relieving cough and sore throat.

Ingredients:

- 1/4 cup fresh ginger, grated

- 1 cup water

- 1/2 cup honey

Instructions:

1. Boil water and add grated ginger. Simmer for 10 minutes, then let it cool.

2. Strain and mix the liquid with honey.

3. Take 1 teaspoon every few hours as needed for cough relief. Store in a jar in the refrigerator for up to a week.

---

3. Ginger Tonic for Immune Support

This drink can help boost immunity, especially during cold and flu season.

Ingredients:

- 1 tablespoon fresh ginger, grated

- Juice of half a lemon

- 1/2 teaspoon turmeric powder (optional, for added benefits)

- A pinch of cayenne pepper (optional, for extra warmth)

- 1 cup warm water

Instructions:

1. Combine all ingredients in a cup.

2. Stir well and drink warm, ideally in the morning.

4. Ginger Bath Soak for Muscle Pain Relief

This ginger bath is soothing for sore muscles and helps ease body aches.

Ingredients:

- 1/4 cup fresh ginger, grated (or 1 tablespoon ginger powder)

- A hot bath

Instructions:

1. Add grated ginger or ginger powder to a muslin cloth or tea bag.

2. Place the bag in the hot bath and let it steep for a few minutes.

3. Soak in the bath for 20-30 minutes to relieve muscle tension and pain.

---

5. Ginger and Lemon Water for Digestion and Weight Loss

This drink boosts metabolism and supports digestion when consumed on an empty stomach.

Ingredients:

- 1-2 inches of fresh ginger, sliced

- Juice of half a lemon

- 1 cup warm water

Instructions:

1. Add ginger slices to warm water and let it steep for 5 minutes.

2. Add lemon juice and stir.

3. Drink first thing in the morning for best results.

6. Ginger Oil for Joint and Muscle Pain Relief

Ginger-infused oil can be used as a massage oil to relieve joint pain and sore muscles.

Ingredients:

- 1/4 cup fresh ginger, grated

- 1/2 cup coconut or olive oil

Instructions:

1. Heat the oil on low and add grated ginger.

2. Let it simmer for about 10 minutes, then cool and strain.

3. Massage onto affected areas for pain relief as needed.

7. Ginger and Garlic Immunity Shot

This potent shot combines ginger and garlic to boost immune health.

Ingredients:

- 1 inch fresh ginger, grated

- 1 garlic clove, minced

- Juice of 1 lemon

- 1/4 teaspoon cayenne pepper (optional, for added warmth)

Instructions:

1. Mix all ingredients together in a small cup.

2. Drink once daily, especially during cold and flu season, to boost immunity.

---

8. Ginger Face Mask for Glowing Skin

This face mask can help rejuvenate and brighten the skin due to ginger's antioxidant properties.

Ingredients:

- 1 teaspoon fresh ginger juice (or 1/2 teaspoon ginger powder)

- 1 tablespoon honey

- 1 teaspoon yogurt (optional, for extra hydration)

Instructions:

1. Mix ginger juice, honey, and yogurt until smooth.

2. Apply the mixture to the face, avoiding the eye area.

3. Leave it on for 10-15 minutes, then rinse with warm water.

9. Ginger and Apple Cider Vinegar Detox Drink

This drink aids digestion and supports detoxification when taken regularly.

Ingredients:

- 1 teaspoon grated ginger
- 1 tablespoon apple cider vinegar
- 1 cup water
- Honey (optional, for taste)

Instructions:

1. Add grated ginger and apple cider vinegar to a cup of water.
2. Stir well, adding honey if desired, and drink in the morning.

10. Ginger Steam Inhalation for Sinus Congestion

This steam inhalation can help relieve sinus congestion and respiratory discomfort.

Ingredients:

- 2 inches of fresh ginger, sliced (or 1 tablespoon ginger powder)

- 4 cups boiling water

Instructions:

1. Add ginger to boiling water, then remove from heat.

2. Lean over the pot, covering your head with a towel, and inhale the steam deeply for 5-10 minutes.

3. Repeat as needed to help clear congestion.

These recipes make use of ginger's versatile medicinal properties, offering natural remedies for digestive health, immune support, respiratory relief, and more.

Common Myths and Misconceptions About Ginger

Ginger, known for its zesty flavor and medicinal properties, has been a staple in kitchens and traditional medicine for centuries. However, its rising popularity has also led to some myths and misconceptions. Let's debunk the most common ones:

---

1. Ginger Cures All Digestive Issues

Myth: Ginger can resolve any and all digestive problems instantly.

Reality: Ginger is effective in easing nausea, bloating, and indigestion, but it is not a cure-all. Chronic digestive issues like acid reflux or IBS require comprehensive medical treatment and lifestyle changes.

2. Consuming Ginger in Any Form Offers the Same Benefits

Myth: Ginger is equally beneficial whether consumed raw, cooked, or dried.

Reality: The form of ginger affects its benefits. Fresh ginger is more effective for nausea and colds, while dried or powdered ginger may be better for inflammation and pain relief. Preparation methods matter!

3. Ginger Has No Side Effects

Myth: Ginger is completely safe in all quantities and situations.

Reality: While ginger is generally safe, excessive consumption can cause heartburn, diarrhea, or irritation in the mouth. People with conditions like gallstones or those taking blood-thinning medications should consume it cautiously.

4. Ginger Can Be Used as a Standalone Cure for Colds

Myth: Ginger alone can completely cure a cold or flu.

Reality: Ginger can alleviate cold symptoms like sore throat and congestion, but it cannot eliminate the root cause of viral infections. It works best as part of a holistic treatment plan, including rest and hydration.

5. Ginger Is Unsafe for Pregnant Women

Myth: Ginger can harm pregnant women and their babies.
Reality: Ginger, in moderate amounts, is safe for most pregnant women and can help reduce nausea and morning sickness. However, excessive doses should be avoided, and it's best to consult a doctor.

6. More Ginger Means Faster Results

Myth: Consuming large amounts of ginger enhances its health benefits.
Reality: Overloading on ginger can lead to adverse effects, such as upset stomach or increased risk of bleeding for those on certain medications. Moderation is crucial for reaping its benefits.

7. Ginger Can Be Stored Indefinitely Without Losing Potency

Myth: Ginger retains its medicinal properties forever.
Reality: Fresh ginger gradually loses potency over time, especially if stored improperly. For maximum benefits, use fresh ginger or store it in the freezer for extended use.

8. Ginger Helps Everyone Lose Weight

Myth: Ginger is a miracle spice that guarantees weight loss.
Reality: While ginger may support metabolism and appetite control, it is not a standalone weight-loss solution. A balanced diet and exercise are essential for sustained results.

9. Drinking Ginger Tea Alone Builds Immunity

Myth: A daily cup of ginger tea can make you completely immune to illnesses.
Reality: Ginger supports the immune system by reducing inflammation and boosting circulation, but it cannot make you invincible to all infections. It works best alongside a nutrient-rich diet and a healthy lifestyle.

10. Ginger Works Immediately for Pain Relief

Myth: Applying ginger directly to the skin or consuming it will instantly relieve pain.
Reality: Ginger has anti-inflammatory properties that can reduce pain over time, but it is not a quick fix. Regular use is needed to see significant benefits, especially for chronic conditions like arthritis.

By understanding these myths and misconceptions, you can better harness the true power of ginger. It's a remarkable spice, but like any remedy, it works best when used thoughtfully and in balance.

Chapter 3: Cumin – Digestion Enhancer

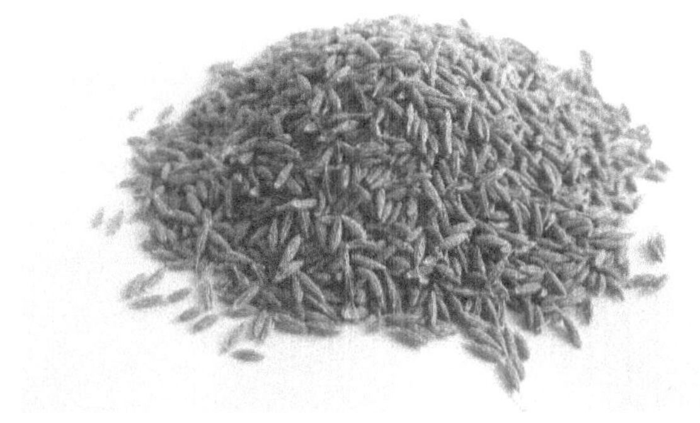

Introduction

Cumin, or *Jeera* in Hindi, is a small, earthy, and aromatic spice that has played an essential role in Indian cooking and traditional medicine for centuries. Derived from the seeds of the *Cuminum cyminum* plant, cumin is well-known for its distinct flavor and ability to enhance the taste of various dishes. Beyond its culinary use, cumin is valued in Ayurveda and traditional medicine for its powerful digestive benefits. Known as a "digestion enhancer," cumin supports gut health, aids in nutrient absorption, and alleviates many common digestive issues.

This chapter explores the medicinal properties of cumin, especially in supporting digestion, improving metabolism, boosting immunity, and more. Cumin's simplicity and effectiveness make it a staple in Indian kitchens, offering a natural way to improve health and well-being through daily cooking.

Medicinal Importance of Cumin

The health benefits of cumin can be attributed to its active compounds, including essential oils, antioxidants, and minerals. Let's explore the specific ways cumin supports various aspects of health.

1. Promotes Digestion and Reduces Bloating

Cumin's primary benefit is its ability to support healthy digestion. It stimulates the production of digestive enzymes, which help break down food and aid in nutrient absorption. Cumin also has carminative properties, meaning it can relieve gas and bloating, making it an effective remedy for indigestion. By enhancing bile production, cumin helps improve the body's ability to digest fats.

- **Home Remedy for Bloating**: Drinking cumin water (jeera water) made by boiling cumin seeds in water can relieve bloating and improve digestion. This drink is especially beneficial when consumed on an empty stomach in the morning.

HEALTH BENEFITS OF CUMIN SEED

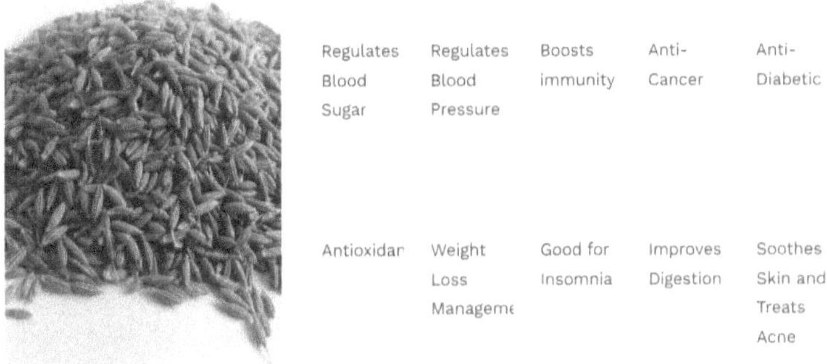

Regulates Blood Sugar	Regulates Blood Pressure	Boosts immunity	Anti-Cancer	Anti-Diabetic
Antioxidar	Weight Loss Manageme	Good for Insomnia	Improves Digestion	Soothes Skin and Treats Acne

2. Natural Remedy for Acid Reflux

Cumin has an alkalizing effect, which helps to reduce acidity in the stomach. By neutralizing stomach acids, cumin can provide relief from acid reflux, heartburn, and other symptoms of acidity. This makes it an excellent remedy for those who experience frequent acid reflux or GERD (gastroesophageal reflux disease).

- **Relief for Acid Reflux**: Chewing a small amount of roasted cumin seeds after meals or drinking cumin-infused water can help balance stomach acidity and prevent heartburn.

3. Enhances Metabolism and Weight Management

Cumin has thermogenic properties, meaning it can increase the body's heat production, thereby boosting metabolism. This can be helpful for weight management, as a faster metabolism can lead to increased calorie burn. Studies have shown that regular consumption of cumin may aid in weight loss, reduce body fat, and improve cholesterol levels.

- **Weight Management Aid**: Drinking cumin water in the morning or adding cumin powder to meals can support metabolism and aid in weight management. It's a low-calorie spice that can be added to almost any dish for added flavor and health benefits.

4. Improves Nutrient Absorption

Cumin contains compounds that help stimulate the release of digestive enzymes, which in turn improves the body's ability to break down and absorb nutrients from food. This is particularly beneficial for those with malabsorption issues or for anyone seeking to maximize the nutritional value of their diet. By aiding in nutrient absorption, cumin helps support overall health and energy levels.

- **Daily Addition to Meals**: Simply incorporating cumin into daily cooking can enhance the body's ability to absorb vitamins, minerals, and other nutrients from food.

5. Rich in Antioxidants

Cumin is a rich source of antioxidants, particularly flavonoids and phenols, which help protect cells from oxidative stress and free radical damage. These antioxidants are crucial for preventing cell damage, supporting healthy aging, and reducing the risk of chronic diseases like cancer and heart disease. The antioxidants in cumin also contribute to skin health by reducing signs of aging.

- **Antioxidant-Rich Drink**: A warm cup of cumin tea made with ground cumin or cumin seeds can be a refreshing and antioxidant-rich beverage to boost overall wellness.

6. Supports Immune Function

Cumin's antimicrobial, antibacterial, and antifungal properties make it a natural immune booster. By helping to fight off infections, cumin can support the body's defense system and reduce the risk of illness. Its high content of iron, vitamin C, and other immune-supporting nutrients makes it a valuable spice for daily use, especially during cold and flu season.

- **Immunity-Boosting Drink**: Cumin, when combined with a pinch of turmeric in warm water, can create an immunity-boosting drink that helps fight off infections and supports the immune system.

7. Helps Regulate Blood Sugar Levels

Studies have indicated that cumin may have anti-diabetic effects, helping to regulate blood sugar levels and improve insulin sensitivity. This makes cumin particularly beneficial for individuals with type 2 diabetes or those at risk of developing it. By helping to control blood sugar levels, cumin can also help reduce cravings and support energy levels throughout the day.

- **Blood Sugar Control**: Drinking cumin water in the morning can help regulate blood sugar levels. Adding cumin powder to food can also help prevent blood sugar spikes after meals.

8. Improves Respiratory Health

Cumin has expectorant properties, which means it can help loosen mucus in the airways, making it easier to expel. This is especially beneficial for those with respiratory issues such as asthma, bronchitis, or chronic cough. Cumin's antibacterial and anti-inflammatory properties also help soothe respiratory inflammation and fight off respiratory infections.

- **Respiratory Relief**: Cumin tea, with a touch of honey and black pepper, can help clear congestion and improve breathing. Adding cumin seeds to soups and broths can also be helpful for respiratory health.

9. Supports Heart Health

Cumin can help improve heart health by reducing cholesterol levels, lowering blood pressure, and improving circulation. Its anti-inflammatory properties reduce inflammation in the blood vessels, which may help prevent the development of heart disease. Cumin's ability to improve lipid profiles and reduce LDL cholesterol is particularly beneficial for those with high cholesterol.

- **Heart-Healthy Drink**: A daily dose of cumin water or adding cumin to meals can help support heart health and maintain healthy cholesterol levels.

10. Promotes Skin Health

Cumin's antioxidant and antimicrobial properties make it beneficial for skin health. It helps fight off skin infections, reduces signs of aging, and promotes a clear, healthy complexion. Cumin is also a source of vitamin E, which supports skin regeneration and repair. Its detoxifying properties help in clearing out impurities from the body, leading to clearer skin.

- **Skin-Glow Remedy**: Drinking cumin-infused water regularly or applying a paste of cumin powder mixed with honey and lemon juice can improve skin health. Additionally, cumin can be added to face masks for a natural glow.

Using Cumin in Daily Life

Cumin is an extremely versatile spice that can easily be incorporated into a wide range of dishes. Here are a few simple ways to use cumin daily:

- **Cumin Water**: Boil one teaspoon of cumin seeds in a cup of water, strain, and drink it in the morning on an empty stomach to improve digestion, boost immunity, and support metabolism.

- **In Cooking**: Add cumin seeds or ground cumin to curries, soups, rice dishes, and marinades to enhance flavor and health benefits.

- **Cumin Paste**: Create a paste by grinding cumin seeds with water. This paste can be applied topically to soothe skin issues or mixed with honey and consumed as a natural remedy.

Ayurvedic Context of Cumin

Cumin (*Cuminum cyminum*), known as *Jeera* in Sanskrit, holds a prominent place in Ayurveda as a powerful digestive and medicinal spice. With its distinctive earthy flavor and aromatic fragrance, cumin has been an integral part of Ayurvedic treatments and Indian cuisine for thousands of years. Ayurveda considers cumin a vital herb for promoting digestive health, balancing doshas, and supporting overall well-being.

Dosha Balancing Properties

In Ayurveda, cumin is primarily known for its ability to pacify *Vata* and *Kapha* doshas, while mildly increasing *Pitta* due to its warming (*ushna*) energy. Its pungent (*katu*) and bitter (*tikta*) taste, combined with its light (*laghu*) and dry (*ruksha*) qualities, make it an effective remedy for digestive disorders, sluggish metabolism, and respiratory ailments.

By balancing *Vata*, cumin helps alleviate gas, bloating, and irregular bowel movements, while its action on *Kapha* aids in clearing mucus, reducing congestion, and stimulating metabolic activity.

Digestive Aid and Appetite Stimulant

Cumin is highly revered in Ayurveda for its digestive properties (*deepana* and *pachana*). It stimulates the secretion of digestive enzymes, enhances the absorption of nutrients, and promotes healthy gut function. Drinking cumin water or adding roasted cumin powder to meals can improve digestion, alleviate bloating, and reduce flatulence. In traditional Ayurvedic practice, a simple infusion of cumin, coriander, and fennel seeds is often prescribed to soothe the digestive tract and support healthy metabolism.

Detoxification and Cleansing

Cumin is considered a natural detoxifier (*ama pachaka*) that helps eliminate toxins (*ama*) from the body. Its cleansing properties support liver function and promote the healthy elimination of waste. Ayurvedic practitioners often recommend cumin-infused water during detoxification routines to purify the blood, enhance kidney function, and promote overall vitality.

Respiratory and Immune Support

Cumin's warming and antimicrobial properties make it an effective remedy for respiratory health. It helps to clear congestion, reduce coughs, and relieve symptoms of colds and flu. A traditional Ayurvedic remedy involves boiling cumin seeds with ginger and honey to create a soothing tea that strengthens the immune system and alleviates respiratory discomfort.

Women's Health and Hormonal Balance

Cumin is often used in Ayurveda to support women's reproductive health. It is believed to regulate menstrual cycles, reduce menstrual cramps, and enhance lactation in nursing mothers. Its warming and carminative properties help to balance hormones and promote overall reproductive wellness.

In Ayurvedic tradition, cumin is more than a spice—it is a versatile healer that supports digestive health, balances doshas, and aids in detoxification, making it a staple in the holistic approach to wellness.

Precautions

While cumin is safe for most people, consuming it in excess may lead to mild digestive discomfort, such as heartburn. Pregnant women and individuals with certain health conditions should consult a healthcare provider before taking cumin supplements, as it may interact with medications or affect certain conditions.

Conclusion

Cumin's ability to enhance digestion and promote overall health makes it an invaluable spice in both cooking and natural medicine. From aiding in digestion and boosting immunity to supporting heart health and improving skin, cumin's medicinal properties are numerous and far-reaching. With its accessibility and ease of use, cumin continues to be a trusted and essential part of traditional Indian kitchens and wellness practices. Adding cumin to daily meals can be a simple yet powerful way to support your health naturally, tapping into centuries-old wisdom with every sprinkle.

<u>RECIPES</u>

Here are **10 medicinal recipes featuring cumin**, a powerhouse spice known for its digestive, anti-inflammatory, and antioxidant properties. These recipes are simple, effective, and rooted in traditional health remedies.

1. Cumin Digestive Tea

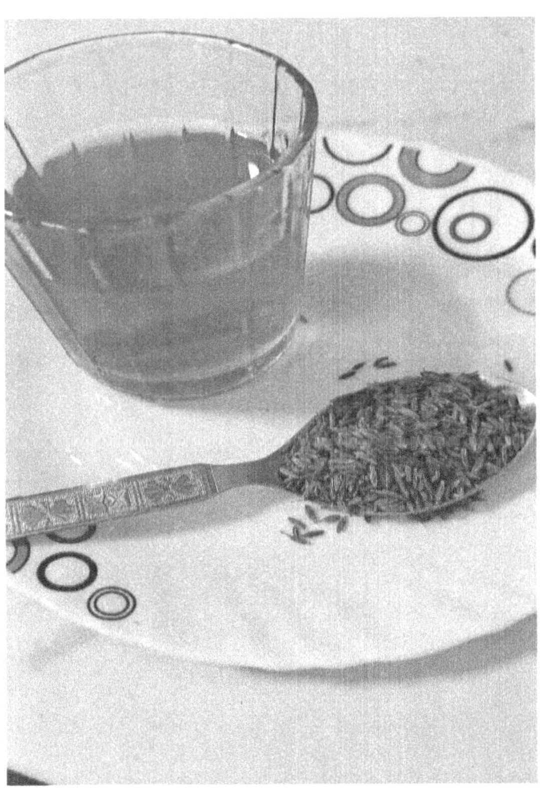

A soothing tea for digestion and bloating.

Ingredients:

- 1 teaspoon cumin seeds
- 1 cup water
- A pinch of ginger (optional)

Instructions:

1. Boil water and add cumin seeds.
2. Simmer for 5 minutes, strain, and enjoy warm.

Benefits: Relieves indigestion, reduces bloating, and soothes the stomach.

This light and aromatic tea provides a natural way to improve digestive comfort, making it a great addition to daily wellness routines.

2. Cumin Water for Weight Loss and Detoxification

Drinking cumin water first thing in the morning may boost metabolism, assist in weight management, and support liver detox.

Ingredients:

- 1 tablespoon cumin seeds

- 1 cup water

- Optional: lemon juice or honey for taste

Instructions:

1. Soak the cumin seeds in water overnight.

2. In the morning, bring the water and cumin seeds to a gentle boil for 2-3 minutes.

3. Strain and drink it warm on an empty stomach.

4. Add a few drops of lemon juice or a touch of honey if desired.

3. Cumin and Ginger Infusion for Cough and Cold Relief

This drink combines cumin with ginger for its antibacterial and anti-inflammatory benefits, helping relieve symptoms of cold and sore throat.

Ingredients:

- 1 teaspoon cumin seeds
- 1 small piece of fresh ginger (or 1/2 teaspoon ground ginger)
- 2 cups water
- Honey (optional)

Instructions:

1. Boil water in a pot and add cumin seeds and ginger.
2. Let it simmer for about 10 minutes, allowing the ingredients to infuse.
3. Strain into a cup and add honey to taste.
4. Drink twice daily for relief from respiratory symptoms.

---

4. Cumin Face Pack for Acne-Prone Skin

Cumin's antibacterial and anti-inflammatory properties make it effective for skin health, especially for treating acne and brightening the complexion.

Ingredients:

- 1 teaspoon cumin powder

- 1 tablespoon honey (or aloe vera gel)

- 1 teaspoon turmeric powder (optional, for extra antibacterial effects)

Instructions:

1. In a small bowl, mix cumin powder, honey (or aloe vera gel), and turmeric powder until a paste forms.

2. Apply the mixture to clean skin, focusing on acne-prone or inflamed areas.

3. Leave it on for 10-15 minutes, then rinse off with lukewarm water.

4. Use 1-2 times per week to help reduce acne and brighten the skin.

---

5. Cumin and Black Pepper Remedy for Boosting Immunity

This mix, taken with honey, provides antioxidants and anti-inflammatory effects, supporting immune health.

Ingredients:

- 1/2 teaspoon cumin powder

- 1/4 teaspoon black pepper powder

- 1 tablespoon honey

Instructions:

1. Mix cumin powder and black pepper powder into the honey until well-blended.

2. Take this mixture once daily, preferably in the morning, to support immunity and reduce inflammation.

6. Cumin Milk for Insomnia and Relaxation

Cumin, when combined with warm milk, can have calming effects, helping with relaxation and sleep.

Ingredients:

- 1/2 teaspoon cumin powder (or 1 teaspoon cumin seeds)

- 1 cup milk (dairy or plant-based)

- Honey or a pinch of nutmeg (optional, for added flavor)

Instructions:

1. Heat the milk and add cumin powder (or crushed cumin seeds).

2. Simmer for a few minutes, allowing the cumin to infuse into the milk.

3. Strain into a cup and add honey or nutmeg, if desired.

4. Drink 30 minutes before bed to promote restful sleep.

7. Cumin-Yogurt Digestive Aid

A cooling remedy for indigestion and acid reflux.

Ingredients:

- 1 cup plain yogurt

- 1/2 teaspoon roasted cumin powder

- A pinch of black salt

Instructions:

1. Mix cumin powder and black salt into yogurt.

2. Eat after meals for better digestion.

Benefits: Reduces acidity, aids digestion, and cools the stomach.

---

8. Cumin-Laced Soup

A nourishing soup for cold relief and digestion.

Ingredients:

- 2 cups vegetable or chicken broth

- 1 teaspoon cumin seeds

- 1/2 teaspoon turmeric powder

Instructions:

1. Simmer broth with cumin seeds and turmeric for 10 minutes.

2. Strain and serve warm.

Benefits: Relieves cold symptoms and soothes digestive discomfort.

---

9. Cumin-Coriander Herbal Blend

A homemade spice mix to balance digestion.

Ingredients:

- 1 tablespoon cumin seeds
- 1 tablespoon coriander seeds
- 1/2 tablespoon fennel seeds

Instructions:

1. Dry roast the seeds and grind into a fine powder.
2. Add a pinch to warm water and drink after meals.

Benefits: Improves digestion, reduces bloating, and cools the stomach.

---

10. Cumin-Infused Oil for Massage

A natural remedy for joint pain and muscle relaxation.

Ingredients:

- 1/4 cup sesame or coconut oil
- 1 teaspoon cumin seeds

Instructions:

1. Warm oil and add cumin seeds.

2. Strain and use for massaging sore areas.

Benefits: Reduces inflammation and improves blood circulation.

---

11. Cumin Herbal Steam

An aromatic therapy for respiratory health.

Ingredients:

- 1 teaspoon cumin seeds

- 4 cups boiling water

Instructions:

1. Add cumin seeds to boiling water.

2. Inhale the steam under a towel for 5–10 minutes.

Benefits: Clears sinuses, soothes respiratory passages, and reduces congestion.

---

12. Cumin Seed Tonic

A quick pick-me-up for digestion and energy.

Ingredients:

- 1 teaspoon cumin seeds

- 1 cup warm water

- A pinch of black salt

Instructions:

1. Boil water, add cumin seeds, and let steep for 5 minutes.

2. Strain, add black salt, and drink warm.

Benefits: Boosts metabolism, relieves nausea, and energizes the body.

These cumin-based recipes are easy to prepare and provide a natural way to enhance digestion, immunity, and overall health. Incorporate them into your routine to experience the healing power of cumin!

Common Myths and Misconceptions About Cumin

Cumin is a cherished spice known for its earthy aroma and medicinal properties, especially for digestion. However, it has also become the subject of myths and misconceptions over time. Let's separate the facts from the myths:

1. Cumin Cures All Digestive Problems Instantly

Myth: A pinch of cumin can resolve all digestive issues immediately.

Reality: While cumin is excellent for improving digestion and reducing bloating, it works best as part of a balanced diet. Chronic conditions like IBS or GERD require medical advice and cannot be resolved solely by cumin.

2. Cumin Can Cause Significant Weight Loss on Its Own

Myth: Consuming cumin daily will lead to dramatic weight loss.

Reality: Cumin can support weight management by boosting metabolism and improving digestion, but it is not a miracle solution. Weight loss requires a combination of diet, exercise, and lifestyle changes.

3. More Cumin Means Better Results

Myth: Adding large amounts of cumin to meals or drinks enhances its health benefits.

Reality: Excessive cumin consumption can cause adverse effects like heartburn, nausea, or low blood sugar levels. Moderate use is key to enjoying its benefits safely.

4. Cumin is Only Good for Digestion

Myth: Cumin's health benefits are limited to aiding digestion.

Reality: Cumin offers numerous benefits beyond digestion, including antioxidant properties, boosting immunity, regulating blood sugar levels, and supporting respiratory health.

5. Cumin Is Only Used in Indian Cuisine

Myth: Cumin is exclusively a part of Indian cooking.

Reality: While cumin is a staple in Indian cuisine, it is widely used in Middle Eastern, Mexican, and Mediterranean dishes. It is a globally loved spice with versatile uses.

6. Cumin Water Is a Cure-All Remedy

Myth: Drinking cumin water daily can cure all ailments.

Reality: Cumin water is beneficial for digestion, detoxification, and hydration, but it cannot cure all health problems. It should complement a healthy diet and lifestyle, not replace them.

7. Cumin Is Unsafe During Pregnancy

Myth: Cumin consumption can harm pregnant women and their babies.

Reality: In moderate amounts, cumin is safe and can even help alleviate nausea and bloating during pregnancy. However, excessive consumption should be avoided, and pregnant women should consult their doctor if unsure.

8. Cumin Causes Dehydration

Myth: Cumin has diuretic properties that can lead to dehydration.

Reality: While cumin may have mild diuretic effects, it is unlikely to cause dehydration when consumed in typical dietary amounts. Staying hydrated with water is always important.

9. Cumin Is Only Available as a Spice

Myth: Cumin is only useful in its powdered or seed form.

Reality: Cumin can also be used as an oil or extract for various medicinal and culinary purposes, expanding its applications beyond the kitchen.

10. Cumin Can Be Consumed Without Any Preparation

Myth: Raw cumin seeds or powder are just as effective as cooked or infused cumin.

Reality: Roasting or lightly cooking cumin seeds enhances their flavor and releases beneficial oils. Cumin water or tea makes its active compounds more accessible for medicinal use.

By debunking these myths, we can fully appreciate cumin as a versatile, health-enhancing spice that plays a vital role in both traditional and modern wellness practices.

Chapter 4: Coriander – The Cooling Healer

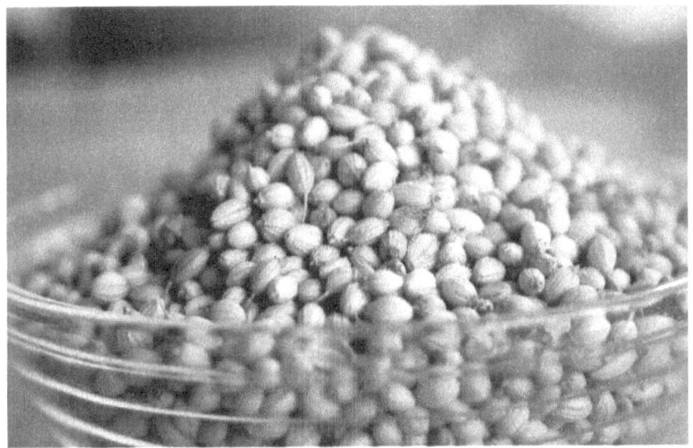

Introduction

Coriander, known as *Dhaniya* in Hindi, is a fragrant and versatile herb and spice with a long-standing role in Indian cuisine and traditional medicine. Coriander comes from the *Coriandrum sativum* plant and offers multiple uses: its leaves, known as cilantro, are used fresh, while its seeds are dried and used as a spice. This small, earthy seed is valued for its cooling properties and digestive benefits, making it a popular ingredient in various cuisines worldwide. However, coriander's medicinal benefits go far beyond flavor – it's a powerful anti-inflammatory, digestive aid, and detoxifying agent.

This chapter explores the many medicinal properties of coriander, particularly in cooling the body, aiding digestion, promoting detoxification, and supporting overall health. Easy to incorporate into daily meals, coriander is a key part of the spice arsenal that brings both flavor and health benefits.

Medicinal Importance of Coriander

Coriander contains bioactive compounds such as linalool, camphor, and antioxidants like quercetin and tocopherols, which contribute to its various health benefits. Here's a closer look at how coriander can promote wellness:

1. Cooling and Detoxifying Effect

Coriander is known for its natural cooling properties, which help to reduce internal heat and calm the body. This makes it an ideal spice for individuals with a tendency toward excess heat or inflammatory conditions. Coriander seeds are particularly effective in promoting detoxification by helping the body expel toxins through the urinary system. In Ayurvedic practices, coriander is often used to balance "pitta" dosha (heat-related imbalances), providing relief from heat and inflammation.

- **Cooling Coriander Water**: Soaking a teaspoon of coriander seeds overnight in water, then drinking it on an empty stomach in the morning, can help cool the body and flush out toxins.

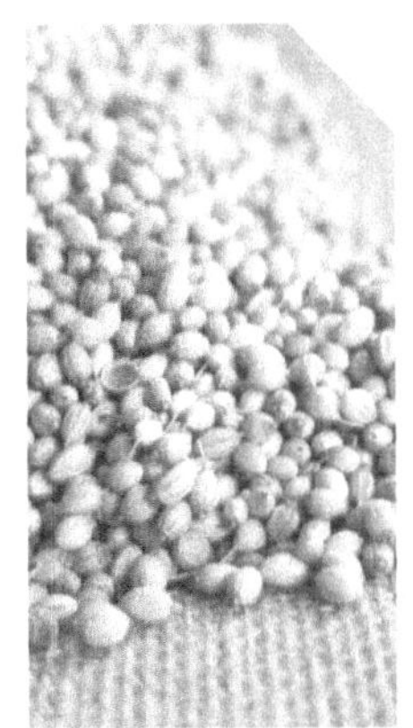

HEALTH BENEFITS OF CORIANDER

Lowers Blood Sugar

Help with stress

Boosts immunity

Reduces cholesterol

Anti-Diabetic

Nourishes your Eye

Good for Hearth Health

Aids in Digestion

Enhances Skin Health

2. Digestive Health and Relief from Bloating

Coriander is an excellent digestive aid, with carminative properties that help relieve gas, bloating, and other digestive discomforts. It stimulates the production of digestive enzymes and promotes the secretion of bile, which assists in breaking down food more effectively. Coriander's fiber content also aids in digestion and prevents constipation.

- **Bloating Relief Drink**: Boiling coriander seeds in water and drinking it as a warm tea can reduce gas and bloating. Adding a pinch of rock salt can further enhance its effectiveness.

3. Anti-Inflammatory Benefits

Coriander is packed with anti-inflammatory compounds that help soothe inflammation and pain in the body. Its antioxidants, such as quercetin and vitamin C, combat free radicals, reducing oxidative stress and helping to prevent chronic inflammation. This anti-inflammatory action is beneficial for managing conditions like arthritis, as it alleviates pain and reduces joint swelling.

- **Natural Remedy for Joint Pain**: Consuming coriander tea or adding coriander powder to meals can help alleviate inflammation. Coriander oil applied topically to sore joints may also provide relief from inflammation.

4. Regulates Blood Sugar Levels

Coriander has been found to support healthy blood sugar levels by enhancing insulin activity and lowering blood glucose levels. This makes coriander particularly beneficial for individuals with diabetes or those at risk of developing type 2 diabetes. Its ability to improve insulin sensitivity and regulate glucose levels can be helpful for managing diabetes naturally.

- **Blood Sugar Regulation**: Drinking coriander seed water or adding coriander powder to meals can support blood sugar balance. A paste of ground coriander seeds and water can also be applied to food as a garnish for additional health benefits.

5. Supports Heart Health

The antioxidants, dietary fiber, and essential minerals in coriander contribute to heart health. Coriander can help lower LDL (bad) cholesterol levels while increasing HDL (good) cholesterol levels, reducing the risk of atherosclerosis and heart disease. Additionally, coriander's anti-inflammatory properties help reduce blood pressure and improve circulation, which further supports cardiovascular health.

- **Heart-Healthy Tip**: Incorporating coriander seeds or powder in daily cooking, especially in soups and curries, can help protect heart health. Drinking coriander water is another simple way to support a healthy heart.

6. Enhances Immunity

Coriander has antimicrobial, antifungal, and antibacterial properties that help the body defend against infections. Rich in vitamin C, vitamin A, and other essential nutrients, coriander strengthens the immune system and helps prevent common illnesses like colds and flu. By eliminating harmful bacteria and pathogens, coriander supports a robust immune response.

- **Immunity-Boosting Drink**: Drinking coriander tea or adding coriander leaves to juices and smoothies can provide a natural boost to the immune system. Fresh coriander can also be incorporated into salads and chutneys to enhance immune strength.

7. Promotes Skin Health

Coriander's detoxifying and antioxidant-rich properties make it an effective remedy for maintaining clear, healthy skin. It helps remove toxins from the body, reducing the appearance of acne, blemishes, and other skin issues. The vitamin E in coriander promotes skin repair and protects against signs of aging. Coriander also has cooling properties that can soothe skin irritations and reduce inflammation in cases of eczema or rashes.

- **Skin-Glow Face Pack**: A paste of ground coriander seeds mixed with honey or yogurt can be applied as a face mask to reduce acne and improve skin tone. Drinking coriander water also supports skin health from the inside out.

8. Supports Urinary Health

Coriander has mild diuretic properties, which help increase urine production and cleanse the urinary system. This can help prevent and manage urinary tract infections (UTIs) by flushing out bacteria and other harmful substances from the body. In traditional medicine, coriander is often recommended for promoting kidney health and preventing fluid retention.

- **Urinary Health Remedy**: Drinking coriander-infused water daily or consuming coriander seeds can help keep the urinary system clear and reduce the risk of infections.

9. Relieves Menstrual Pain

Coriander's anti-inflammatory and antispasmodic properties make it useful for relieving menstrual cramps and discomfort. By relaxing the muscles and reducing inflammation, coriander can help alleviate the pain associated with menstruation. Its cooling effect also helps balance excess heat and reduce irritability during the menstrual cycle.

- **Menstrual Cramp Relief**: Drinking coriander seed water or consuming coriander leaves with honey can be a natural remedy for menstrual discomfort.

10. Supports Healthy Vision

Rich in vitamin A and other antioxidants, coriander promotes eye health and helps protect against age-related macular degeneration and other vision problems. The vitamin C in coriander also plays a role in reducing oxidative stress, which can impact eye health. Regular consumption of coriander can support clear vision and maintain eye health.

- **Eye Health Tip**: Including fresh coriander leaves in your diet or drinking coriander seed water can provide essential nutrients for healthy eyes.

Incorporating Coriander into Daily Life

Coriander can be used in many ways, making it easy to include in daily meals and drinks. Here are some practical ways to add coriander to your routine:

- **Coriander Water**: Soak a teaspoon of coriander seeds in water overnight, strain, and drink it in the morning on an empty stomach for detoxification and digestive support.

- **Cooking**: Add ground coriander or whole seeds to curries, soups, and stews to enhance flavor and health benefits. Fresh coriander leaves make an excellent garnish for any dish.

- **Coriander Tea**: Boil coriander seeds in water, strain, and drink as a warm tea to relieve bloating, aid digestion, and support overall wellness.

92

Ayurvedic Context of Coriander

Coriander (*Coriandrum sativum*), known as *Dhanyaka* in Sanskrit, is a cherished herb in Ayurveda, celebrated for its cooling, soothing, and balancing properties. Both the seeds and leaves (commonly known as cilantro) are used extensively in Ayurvedic medicine and Indian cuisine. Revered as a powerful digestive aid and detoxifier, coriander is regarded as a "tridoshic" herb, meaning it can balance all three doshas—*Vata*, *Pitta*, and *Kapha*—making it a versatile and indispensable ingredient in holistic health practices.

Dosha Balancing Properties

Coriander's primary taste is mild and slightly bitter (*tikta*), with sweet (*madhura*) and astringent (*kashaya*) undertones. It has a cooling (*sheeta*) energy and a light (*laghu*) quality, which makes it particularly effective in balancing *Pitta* dosha by reducing heat and inflammation in the body. Additionally, it helps to alleviate *Vata*-related digestive issues such as bloating and gas, and its lightness can moderate the sluggishness associated with *Kapha*.

This unique ability to balance all three doshas makes coriander an essential herb for maintaining overall harmony and equilibrium in the body.

Digestive and Metabolic Support

Coriander is highly valued in Ayurveda for its digestive properties (*deepana* and *pachana*). It stimulates the secretion of digestive enzymes, enhances appetite, and promotes the efficient assimilation of nutrients. Coriander seeds are often brewed into a tea or infused in water to soothe the digestive system, relieve indigestion, and reduce acidity. It is also an effective remedy for relieving bloating, flatulence, and nausea, especially when combined with cumin and fennel.

Detoxification and Purification

Coriander is considered a natural detoxifier (*ama pachaka*) that supports the body's natural cleansing processes. It helps to eliminate toxins (*ama*), purify the blood, and promote healthy liver function. In Ayurvedic detox routines, coriander seed water is often recommended to flush out impurities, enhance kidney function, and promote healthy skin.

Cooling and Anti-Inflammatory Properties

Due to its cooling nature, coriander is frequently used to soothe inflammatory conditions and reduce excess heat in the body. It is beneficial for conditions such as acid reflux, skin rashes, and urinary tract infections. Coriander juice, mixed with a pinch of rock salt, is a traditional Ayurvedic remedy for cooling the body and calming inflammation.

Respiratory and Immune Support

Coriander's antimicrobial and anti-inflammatory properties also make it beneficial for respiratory health. It helps to clear congestion, alleviate coughs, and soothe sore throats.

Coriander tea, infused with honey and ginger, is a common Ayurvedic remedy for respiratory discomfort and boosting immunity.

In Ayurveda, coriander is not just a spice but a holistic healer, promoting digestion, detoxification, and overall balance, making it a vital herb in the pursuit of optimal health and well-being.

Precautions

While coriander is generally safe for consumption, some people may experience allergic reactions. Excessive consumption may also lower blood pressure significantly. Pregnant women and individuals on blood pressure-lowering medications should consult a healthcare provider before using coriander as a supplement.

Conclusion

Coriander's cooling, digestive, and detoxifying properties make it a powerful addition to the kitchen and an essential spice for natural healing. From promoting digestion and heart health to supporting immunity and clear skin, coriander offers a range of medicinal benefits. Adding coriander to meals is a simple and effective way to harness the spice's healing powers, creating a balanced, health-promoting diet with roots in ancient practices. As a humble but potent spice, coriander truly lives up to its reputation as a cooling healer, making it an indispensable part of daily wellness.

<u>RECIPES</u>

1. Coriander Seed Tea for Digestion and Detoxification

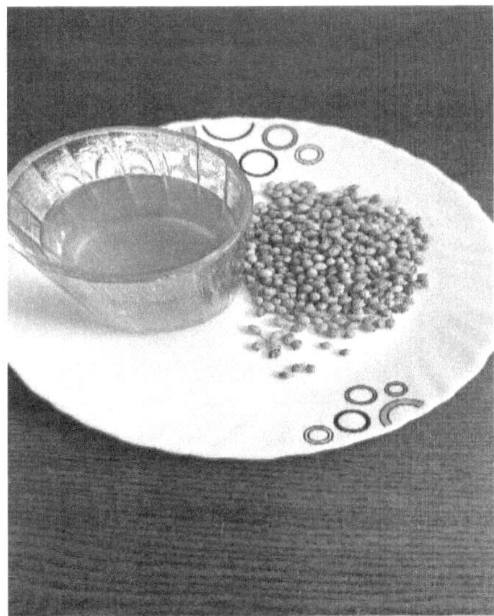

This tea helps relieve digestive discomfort, reduce bloating, and supports gentle detoxification.

Ingredients:

- 1 teaspoon coriander seeds

- 1 cup water

- Optional: a pinch of fennel seeds (for extra digestive benefits)

Instructions:

1. Boil the water and add the coriander seeds (and fennel seeds, if using).

2. Let it simmer for about 5 minutes.

3. Strain and drink warm, preferably after meals, to soothe digestion and aid in detoxification.

2. Coriander Water for Weight Loss and Detox

Drinking coriander-infused water in the morning can boost metabolism, assist with weight management, and support liver health.

Ingredients:

- 1 tablespoon coriander seeds
- 1 cup water

Instructions:

1. Soak coriander seeds in water overnight.
2. In the morning, strain and drink the water on an empty stomach.
3. Repeat daily for 1-2 weeks for best results.

---

3. Coriander and Honey Remedy for Cough and Cold

Coriander seeds, combined with honey, can help reduce congestion, relieve cough, and improve respiratory health.

Ingredients:

- 1 teaspoon crushed coriander seeds
- 1 tablespoon honey

Instructions:

1. Crush the coriander seeds and mix them with honey.

2. Take this mixture 1-2 times daily to relieve cold symptoms and soothe the throat.

4. Coriander Seed Water for Blood Sugar Control

This simple drink, taken regularly, may help regulate blood sugar levels, making it beneficial for people with diabetes.

Ingredients:

- 1 tablespoon coriander seeds

- 1 cup water

Instructions:

1. Soak coriander seeds in water overnight.

2. Strain and drink this water in the morning on an empty stomach.

3. Repeat daily for blood sugar support (consult a doctor before starting if on medication).

5. Coriander Leaf Juice for Skin Health and Detoxification

Coriander leaf juice, with its antibacterial and anti-inflammatory properties, helps cleanse the skin, reduce acne, and support internal detox.

Ingredients:

- 1/2 cup fresh coriander leaves

- 1/2 cup water

- Optional: a squeeze of lemon or a pinch of turmeric (for added skin benefits)

Instructions:

1. Blend coriander leaves with water until smooth.

2. Strain, add lemon juice or turmeric if desired, and drink immediately.

3. Consume regularly to promote clear skin and support detox.

---

6. Coriander and Ginger Infusion for Anti-Inflammatory Benefits

This drink combines coriander and ginger, two potent anti-inflammatory agents, which may benefit people with arthritis or other inflammatory conditions.

Ingredients:

- 1 teaspoon coriander seeds

- 1 small piece of ginger (or 1/2 teaspoon ground ginger)

- 1 cup water

Instructions:

1. Boil water and add coriander seeds and ginger.

2. Simmer for 10 minutes, then strain into a cup.

3. Drink once daily to help reduce inflammation and joint pain.

7. Coriander Face Mask for Acne and Bright Skin

This face mask utilizes coriander's antibacterial properties to reduce acne and brighten the skin.

Ingredients:

- 1 tablespoon coriander leaves (crushed or blended)

- 1 tablespoon yogurt (for soothing and moisturizing)

- A pinch of turmeric powder (optional, for extra antibacterial effects)

Instructions:

1. Mix crushed coriander leaves with yogurt and turmeric to form a paste.

2. Apply to clean skin and leave on for 15-20 minutes.

3. Rinse off with warm water. Use once or twice a week for clearer skin.

8. Coriander-Infused Oil for Muscle and Joint Pain

Coriander seed oil has anti-inflammatory properties and can be used as a massage oil for relief from sore muscles and joint pain.

Ingredients:

- 1 tablespoon coriander seeds

- 1/2 cup olive or coconut oil

Instructions:

1. Heat the oil on low and add the coriander seeds.

2. Let it simmer for 10 minutes, then remove from heat and cool.

3. Strain and store the infused oil in a glass jar.

4. Massage onto sore muscles or joints as needed.

---

9. Coriander and Mint Drink for Cooling and Hydration

This refreshing drink is great for cooling the body, hydrating, and reducing heat-related headaches or stomach discomfort.

Ingredients:

- 1/4 cup fresh coriander leaves

- 1/4 cup fresh mint leaves

- 2 cups cold water

- Juice of half a lemon

Instructions:

1. Blend coriander and mint leaves with water and strain.

2. Add lemon juice and serve cold, especially in hot weather or after a workout.

10. Coriander Honey Remedy

A quick fix for sore throat and inflammation.

Ingredients:

- 1 teaspoon coriander seed powder

- 1 teaspoon honey

Instructions:

1. Mix coriander seed powder with honey into a paste.

2. Take directly twice a day.

Benefits: Soothes sore throat, fights infections, and reduces inflammation.

These medicinal recipes utilize coriander's versatile benefits to support digestion, skin health, detoxification, and pain relief, making it a valuable addition to natural health remedies.

Common Myths and Misconceptions About Coriander

Coriander, loved for its citrusy flavor and versatile use in the kitchen, is a staple in many cuisines. However, myths and misconceptions about its properties and uses can cloud its true benefits. Let's uncover the truth about this incredible herb and spice.

---

1. Coriander and Cilantro Are Completely Different

Myth: Coriander and cilantro are two entirely different plants.
Reality: Coriander and cilantro come from the same plant, *Coriandrum sativum*. In some regions (like the U.S.), "cilantro" refers to the fresh leaves, while "coriander" refers to the seeds. Both share similar health benefits, though they are used differently.

---

2. Coriander Is Only Used for Flavoring

Myth: Coriander has no medicinal value and is only a culinary spice.
Reality: Coriander is packed with medicinal properties, including aiding digestion, detoxifying the body, and regulating blood sugar levels. It is as beneficial for health as it is for enhancing flavor.

---

3. Coriander Causes Allergies in Everyone

Myth: Coriander is highly allergenic and unsafe for sensitive individuals.

Reality: While coriander may trigger allergies in a small number of people, it is generally safe for most. Allergies to coriander are rare compared to other common allergens like nuts or shellfish.

4. Coriander Can Be Used in Unlimited Quantities

Myth: You can consume as much coriander as you want without any side effects.

Reality: Excessive consumption of coriander can sometimes lead to gastrointestinal discomfort, dizziness, or low blood pressure. Like any spice, it should be used in moderation.

5. Coriander Is a Feminine Herb

Myth: Coriander is more beneficial for women and less useful for men.

Reality: Coriander has health benefits for everyone, regardless of gender. It supports hormonal balance, digestion, and detoxification, making it equally valuable for men and women.

6. Cooking Destroys Coriander's Nutritional Value

Myth: Heat eliminates all the health benefits of coriander.
Reality: While cooking may reduce the potency of certain nutrients, coriander still retains significant medicinal properties when cooked. Using coriander seeds and powders in stews, soups, or spice blends remains beneficial.

7. Coriander Detoxifies Everything Instantly

Myth: A single serving of coriander water or tea will instantly detoxify the body.
Reality: Coriander supports detoxification of heavy metals and toxins over time, but it is not a magical or immediate detox solution. Consistent use alongside a healthy lifestyle is necessary for noticeable effects.

8. Coriander Is Only Useful for Digestion

Myth: Coriander's benefits are limited to aiding digestion.
Reality: While coriander is excellent for soothing digestive issues, it also supports healthy skin, boosts immunity, improves heart health, and helps regulate blood sugar levels.

9. Coriander Is Ineffective in Powdered Form

Myth: Coriander powder loses its medicinal properties compared to fresh leaves or whole seeds.
Reality: While freshly ground seeds or leaves may have more flavor and potency, coriander powder still contains many beneficial compounds, especially when stored properly.

10. Coriander Is a "Weak" Herb Compared to Others

Myth: Coriander is less potent than other medicinal herbs and spices.

Reality: Coriander is a powerhouse of antioxidants, anti-inflammatory compounds, and essential nutrients. It may not have the strong pungency of spices like turmeric or ginger, but it offers unique and valuable health benefits.

By busting these myths, we can truly appreciate coriander as a versatile and medicinal ingredient that deserves its place in every kitchen. It's more than just a garnish or seasoning—it's a holistic healer!

Chapter 5: Fenugreek – The Ancient Healer

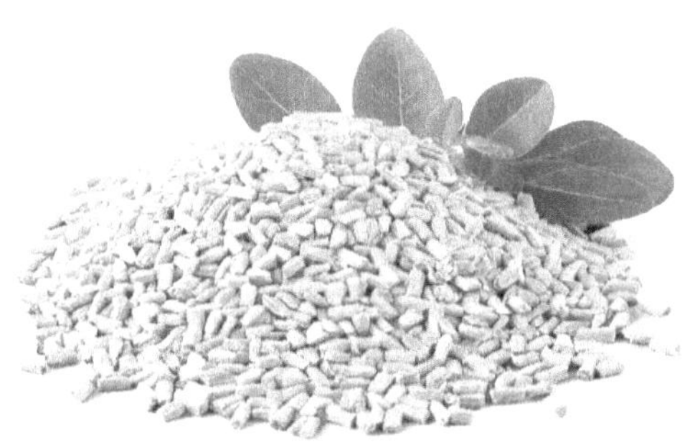

Introduction

Fenugreek, or *Methi* in Hindi, is a unique herb and spice with a long history of medicinal and culinary use, especially in India and the Middle East. Known for its slightly bitter taste and aromatic seeds, fenugreek has a distinctive place in Ayurvedic and traditional medicine. Rich in nutrients and bioactive compounds, it offers a wealth of health benefits, ranging from blood sugar regulation to promoting digestive health and reducing inflammation. Fenugreek is commonly used in both its seed and leaf forms, each bringing valuable properties to various recipes and remedies.

In this chapter, we'll dive into the medicinal benefits of fenugreek, highlighting its significance in maintaining health and managing common ailments. Recognized as a "go-to" spice for promoting overall well-being, fenugreek is easy to incorporate into daily meals or as part of home remedies.

Medicinal Importance of Fenugreek

Fenugreek contains numerous health-boosting compounds, including saponins, flavonoids, fiber, vitamins, and minerals like iron, magnesium, and manganese. These compounds make fenugreek a powerhouse for health, especially in the following areas:

1. Regulates Blood Sugar Levels

Fenugreek is widely regarded for its ability to support healthy blood sugar levels, making it particularly beneficial for individuals with diabetes or those at risk of developing it. The soluble fiber in fenugreek seeds slows down carbohydrate digestion and absorption, leading to more gradual increases in blood sugar levels. Additionally, fenugreek has compounds that may improve insulin sensitivity, making it a valuable aid for blood sugar management.

- **Fenugreek Seed Remedy**: Soaking fenugreek seeds overnight and consuming them on an empty stomach in the morning is a traditional practice for regulating blood sugar levels. You can also add ground fenugreek to foods or drink fenugreek tea as an alternative.

2. Enhances Digestive Health

Fenugreek's high fiber content and ability to soothe the digestive tract make it beneficial for digestive health. It can help relieve constipation, reduce acid reflux, and ease indigestion. The mucilage in fenugreek seeds coats the stomach lining, reducing irritation and promoting a healthy gut. Its slightly bitter taste stimulates the release of digestive enzymes, which supports digestion.

- **Digestive Aid**: Drinking fenugreek tea or soaking fenugreek seeds in water can relieve digestive issues like bloating, gas, and indigestion.

HEALTH BENEFITS OF FENUGREEK

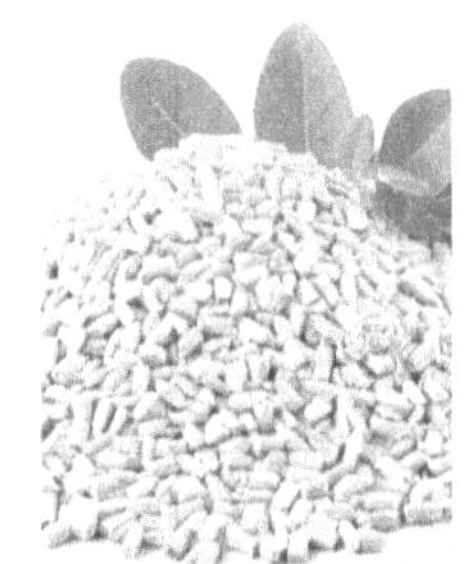

Supports digestion

Lowers blood sugar

Boosts milk production

Reduces inflammation

Improves heart health

Aids weight loss

Relieves menstrual cramps

Enhances skin health

Lowers cholesterol levels

Fights hair loss

3. Reduces Inflammation and Joint Pain

Fenugreek contains anti-inflammatory compounds like diosgenin and flavonoids, which can help reduce inflammation in the body. This property makes it a useful remedy for joint pain and arthritis. By reducing inflammation, fenugreek helps alleviate discomfort and improve mobility, especially in individuals with chronic inflammatory conditions.

- **Joint Pain Remedy**: Applying a paste made from ground fenugreek seeds mixed with warm water or coconut oil to sore joints can provide relief from inflammation and joint pain. Drinking fenugreek tea also provides internal anti-inflammatory benefits.

4. Supports Weight Management

Fenugreek may help support weight management by promoting feelings of fullness and reducing appetite. The high fiber content in fenugreek helps curb hunger, which can be beneficial for individuals looking to manage their weight. Additionally, its effect on blood sugar regulation helps prevent cravings for sugary or high-carb foods, making it easier to maintain a balanced diet.

- **Appetite Suppressant**: Adding fenugreek seeds to meals or drinking fenugreek-infused water before meals can help reduce hunger and support weight management efforts.

5. Improves Heart Health

Fenugreek's cholesterol-lowering properties make it beneficial for heart health. It can help reduce LDL (bad) cholesterol levels, which can lower the risk of heart disease. Fenugreek also has the potential to reduce blood pressure and improve circulation, both of which contribute to cardiovascular wellness.

- **Heart-Healthy Drink**: Drinking fenugreek water daily or incorporating fenugreek seeds into meals may help manage cholesterol levels and support heart health.

6. Boosts Lactation in Nursing Mothers

Fenugreek has traditionally been used to stimulate milk production in nursing mothers. The phytoestrogen compounds in fenugreek, particularly diosgenin, help increase milk supply by mimicking the effects of estrogen. This makes fenugreek a popular herbal remedy for lactating mothers looking to enhance milk flow.

- **Milk Supply Aid**: Consuming fenugreek seeds or fenugreek supplements, after consulting with a healthcare provider, can help improve milk production in breastfeeding mothers.

7. Supports Healthy Skin and Hair

Fenugreek's antioxidant properties and high vitamin C content make it beneficial for skin and hair health. It helps fight oxidative stress, reduces signs of aging, and promotes a clear, glowing complexion. Fenugreek can also be used to treat dandruff, scalp irritation, and hair fall, thanks to its nourishing and anti-inflammatory properties.

- **Skin and Hair Remedy**: A paste made from soaked fenugreek seeds can be applied as a face mask to reduce blemishes and signs of aging. Fenugreek paste applied to the scalp helps treat dandruff and promotes healthy hair growth.

8. Eases Menstrual Cramps and Symptoms of PMS

Fenugreek's natural anti-inflammatory and analgesic properties make it useful for relieving menstrual cramps and symptoms of premenstrual syndrome (PMS). The compounds in fenugreek help relax muscles, reduce inflammation, and alleviate pain associated with menstruation, providing natural relief for menstrual discomfort.

- **Menstrual Pain Relief**: Drinking fenugreek tea or consuming fenugreek seeds can help reduce menstrual cramps. A warm compress using fenugreek water can also provide external relief from menstrual pain.

9. Promotes Respiratory Health

Fenugreek is often used in traditional remedies to alleviate respiratory issues, as it helps loosen mucus and soothe inflammation in the respiratory tract. This makes it beneficial for managing coughs, colds, and symptoms of bronchitis. The antimicrobial properties in fenugreek also help reduce the risk of respiratory infections.

- **Respiratory Remedy**: Drinking fenugreek tea with honey and ginger can help alleviate cough and congestion. Adding a pinch of fenugreek powder to soups or stews can also provide respiratory benefits.

10. Antioxidant Properties for Cellular Health

Fenugreek is rich in antioxidants, which help fight free radicals in the body, protecting cells from oxidative damage. This antioxidant action supports overall health and reduces the risk of chronic diseases like cancer and heart disease. By promoting cellular health, fenugreek also contributes to healthy aging and vitality.

- **Antioxidant-Rich Tea**: Drinking fenugreek tea regularly is an easy way to benefit from its antioxidant properties. Including fenugreek seeds in meals also provides a steady supply of antioxidants.

Incorporating Fenugreek into Daily Life

Fenugreek can be used in multiple ways, making it easy to incorporate into daily health routines. Here are some practical suggestions:

- **Fenugreek Water**: Soak a teaspoon of fenugreek seeds in a glass of water overnight, then strain and drink it on an empty stomach in the morning. This is particularly beneficial for blood sugar regulation and digestion.

- **Cooking**: Fenugreek seeds and leaves can be added to curries, stir-fries, and soups. Ground fenugreek seeds can be used as a seasoning in various dishes to enhance flavor and health benefits.

- **Fenugreek Tea**: Boil fenugreek seeds in water to make a soothing tea, which can help with digestion, inflammation, and respiratory health.

Ayurvedic Context of Fenugreek

Fenugreek (*Trigonella foenum-graecum*), known as *Methi* in Hindi and *Methika* in Sanskrit, holds a prominent place in Ayurvedic medicine as a powerful herb for promoting health and wellness. It is prized for its warming, nourishing, and rejuvenating properties, making it a popular remedy for a variety of ailments. Both the seeds and leaves of fenugreek are utilized in Ayurveda for their medicinal benefits, particularly in balancing doshas, enhancing digestion, and supporting metabolic health.

Dosha Balancing Properties

Fenugreek is primarily known for balancing *Vata* and *Kapha* doshas, thanks to its heating (*ushna*), bitter (*tikta*), and pungent (*katu*) qualities. Its heavy (*guru*) and oily (*snigdha*) nature also make it beneficial for addressing *Vata* imbalances, which are often characterized by dryness, coldness, and irregular digestion. However, due to its heating effect, fenugreek can aggravate *Pitta* when consumed in excess, especially during hot weather or by individuals with a *Pitta* constitution.

Digestive and Metabolic Support

In Ayurveda, fenugreek is highly valued for its ability to stimulate *Agni* (digestive fire) and promote healthy digestion. It is often used to alleviate digestive issues such as bloating, gas, constipation, and loss of appetite. Fenugreek seeds soaked in water overnight and consumed on an empty stomach are a traditional remedy for improving gut health and preventing indigestion.

Fenugreek is also known to support metabolic function and is frequently recommended for managing blood sugar levels. Its seeds contain soluble fiber and compounds that enhance insulin sensitivity, making it a popular Ayurvedic remedy for individuals with diabetes or those seeking to stabilize blood sugar.

Anti-Inflammatory and Joint Health

Fenugreek's anti-inflammatory properties are well-regarded in Ayurveda, where it is used to alleviate joint pain, muscle stiffness, and arthritis-related inflammation. A paste made from fenugreek seeds and warm water is often applied topically to reduce swelling and relieve pain. Internally, fenugreek tea or a decoction can help manage chronic inflammatory conditions.

Women's Health and Hormonal Balance

Fenugreek is considered a tonic for women's health in Ayurveda. It is commonly used to regulate menstrual cycles, reduce menstrual cramps, and support lactation in nursing mothers due to its galactagogue properties. Fenugreek seeds are often consumed with warm milk or ghee to enhance reproductive health and hormonal balance.

Detoxification and Immunity

Fenugreek's cleansing properties help eliminate toxins (*ama*) from the body, purify the blood, and boost overall immunity. It is often included in detox regimens to support liver health and improve energy levels.

In summary, fenugreek is a versatile Ayurvedic herb that supports digestion, metabolism, joint health, and hormonal balance, making it a valuable addition to a holistic wellness routine.

118

Precautions

While fenugreek is safe for most people, it may cause mild digestive discomfort in some cases if consumed in excess. Pregnant women, individuals on blood-thinning medications, and those with hormone-sensitive conditions should consult a healthcare provider before using fenugreek as a supplement, as it can interact with medications and affect certain conditions.

Conclusion

Fenugreek's range of medicinal benefits makes it a versatile spice with an important place in natural healing. From supporting digestion and blood sugar control to enhancing skin, hair, and heart health, fenugreek offers numerous health advantages that are easily accessible. As a staple in Indian kitchens and traditional medicine, fenugreek continues to be a valuable natural remedy that brings holistic benefits to daily life. With its long history as an ancient healer, fenugreek is truly a testament to the power of nature in promoting wellness and longevity.

<u>RECIPES</u>

Fenugreek seeds are highly valued in traditional medicine for their numerous health benefits, including blood sugar control, digestion improvement, and hormone regulation. Here are some effective medicinal recipes using fenugreek seeds:

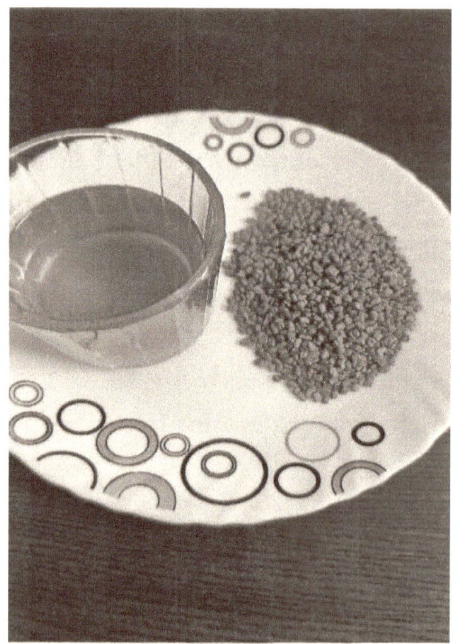

1. Fenugreek Water for Blood Sugar Control

Helps regulate blood sugar and improve insulin sensitivity.

Ingredients:

- 1 tablespoon fenugreek seeds

- 1 cup water

Instructions:

1. Soak fenugreek seeds in water overnight.

2. Strain and drink the water on an empty stomach in the morning.

3. Repeat daily for optimal results.

2. Fenugreek Tea for Digestion

Relieves bloating, indigestion, and promotes a healthy gut.
Ingredients:

- 1 teaspoon fenugreek seed.

- 1 cup water

- A pinch of ginger (optional)

Instructions:

1. Boil water and add fenugreek seeds.

2. Simmer for 5-10 minutes.

3. Strain and drink warm after meals.

3. Fenugreek and Honey Remedy for Sore Throat

Soothes throat irritation and reduces coughing.
Ingredients:

- 1 teaspoon fenugreek powder

- 1 tablespoon honey

Instructions:

1. Mix fenugreek powder with honey to form a paste.

2. Take 1/2 teaspoon of this mixture twice a day for relief.

4. Fenugreek Seeds for Lactation Support

Enhances milk production in breastfeeding mothers.
Ingredients:

- 1 teaspoon fenugreek seeds
- 1 cup milk

Instructions:

1. Boil fenugreek seeds in milk for 5-7 minutes.
2. Strain and drink warm once daily.

---

5. Fenugreek Hair Mask for Hair Growth

Promotes healthy scalp and reduces hair fall.
Ingredients:

- 2 tablespoons fenugreek seeds
- 1/2 cup water
- 2 tablespoons yogurt (optional)

Instructions:

1. Soak fenugreek seeds in water overnight and grind into a paste.
2. Mix with yogurt if desired and apply to the scalp.
3. Leave for 30 minutes, then rinse with water.

6. Fenugreek and Lemon Drink for Weight Loss

Boosts metabolism and aids in fat loss.

Ingredients:

- 1 tablespoon fenugreek seeds
- 1 cup warm water
- Juice of half a lemon

Instructions:

1. Soak fenugreek seeds overnight and strain.
2. Add lemon juice to the water and drink on an empty stomach.

7. Fenugreek Paste for Skin Health

Treats acne, soothes inflammation, and brightens skin.

Ingredients:

- 1 tablespoon fenugreek seeds
- 2 tablespoons water
- A pinch of turmeric (optional)

Instructions:

1. Soak fenugreek seeds for a few hours and grind into a paste.
2. Mix with turmeric and apply to the face.

3. Leave for 15-20 minutes, then rinse off.

---

8. Fenugreek Powder for Cholesterol Management

Helps lower LDL cholesterol and improve heart health.
Ingredients:

- 1 teaspoon fenugreek powder

- 1 cup warm water or milk

Instructions:

1. Mix fenugreek powder into warm water or milk.

2. Drink once daily, preferably in the morning.

---

9. Fenugreek Oil for Joint Pain Relief

Eases inflammation and soothes aching joints.
Ingredients:

- 2 tablespoons fenugreek seeds

- 1/4 cup coconut or sesame oil

Instructions:

1. Heat oil on low and add fenugreek seeds.

2. Simmer for 10 minutes, then strain.

3. Massage the oil onto affected joints as needed.

10. Fenugreek Seeds for Menstrual Cramps

Reduces pain and discomfort during menstruation.
Ingredients:

- 1 teaspoon fenugreek seeds

- 1 cup hot water

Instructions:

1. Soak fenugreek seeds in hot water for 10 minutes.

2. Strain and drink warm during menstrual cramps for relief.

These recipes highlight the versatility of fenugreek seeds in addressing various health concerns naturally. Always consult a healthcare professional if you're using fenugreek as a remedy while on medication or if you have specific health conditions.

Common Myths and Misconceptions About Fenugreek

Fenugreek, a widely used spice in Indian kitchens and herbal medicine, is celebrated for its numerous health benefits. However, it has become surrounded by myths and misconceptions that often distort its true value. Let's clarify the truth about fenugreek:

1. Fenugreek Can Instantly Boost Breast Milk Supply

Myth: Fenugreek guarantees an immediate and dramatic increase in breast milk production for nursing mothers.
Reality: While fenugreek is known to support lactation, its effectiveness varies among individuals. It is not a guaranteed solution, and adequate hydration, nutrition, and proper breastfeeding techniques are equally important.

2. Fenugreek Is Only for Women

Myth: Fenugreek is primarily a women's herb, useful for hormonal balance and lactation.
Reality: Fenugreek offers health benefits for everyone, regardless of gender. It can improve digestion, boost testosterone levels, regulate blood sugar, and enhance overall vitality in both men and women.

3. Fenugreek Is Unsafe During Pregnancy

Myth: Consuming fenugreek during pregnancy can harm the mother or baby.

Reality: In small, culinary amounts, fenugreek is generally safe during pregnancy. However, excessive intake (especially as a supplement) can cause uterine contractions, so it's best to consult a healthcare provider.

4. Fenugreek Works as a Weight-Loss Miracle

Myth: Regular consumption of fenugreek guarantees rapid weight loss.

Reality: Fenugreek may aid weight management by curbing appetite and improving metabolism, but it is not a magic solution. Sustainable weight loss requires a balanced diet and regular exercise.

5. Fenugreek Leaves and Seeds Have the Same Benefits

Myth: Fenugreek leaves and seeds are interchangeable and provide identical health benefits.

Reality: Both have unique benefits. Fenugreek seeds are rich in fiber, antioxidants, and saponins, while the leaves are high in vitamins, minerals, and iron. They complement each other but serve different purposes.

6. Fenugreek Has No Side Effects

Myth: Fenugreek is completely safe in all quantities and situations.
Reality: Excessive consumption of fenugreek can lead to side effects such as diarrhea, bloating, a maple syrup-like body odor, or low blood sugar levels. Moderation is key.

7. Fenugreek Can Cure Diabetes

Myth: Fenugreek is a standalone cure for diabetes.
Reality: Fenugreek helps regulate blood sugar levels due to its fiber content and ability to improve insulin sensitivity, but it cannot replace medication or a proper diabetes management plan.

8. Fenugreek Can Be Used by Everyone Without Caution

Myth: Fenugreek is universally safe for all individuals.
Reality: People with allergies to legumes, those on blood-thinning medications, or those with hypoglycemia should exercise caution. Always consult a healthcare professional before using it as a supplement.

9. Fenugreek Is Only Beneficial When Eaten

Myth: Fenugreek needs to be consumed to deliver health benefits.

Reality: Fenugreek can also be used topically for skin health, hair growth, and reducing inflammation. It has diverse applications beyond ingestion.

10. Cooking Fenugreek Reduces Its Medicinal Properties

Myth: Heat destroys fenugreek's nutrients and reduces its health benefits.

Reality: Cooking fenugreek may slightly alter its nutrient profile but does not eliminate its medicinal properties. Toasting or lightly cooking the seeds can enhance their flavor and digestibility.

By debunking these myths, we gain a clearer understanding of fenugreek's versatility and true potential. This humble spice is not just a kitchen staple but a powerful ally in promoting health—when used wisely!

Chapter 6: Cinnamon – The Warming Healer

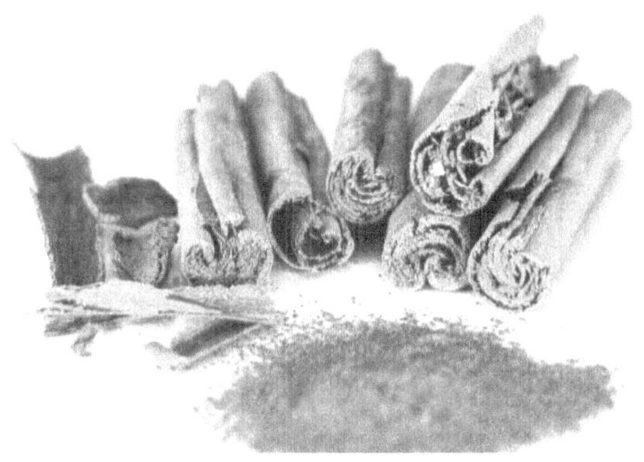

Introduction

Cinnamon, known as *Dalchini* in Hindi, is an ancient spice that has been valued for its warming, aromatic flavor and numerous medicinal benefits. Derived from the inner bark of the *Cinnamomum* tree, cinnamon has a distinctive sweet and spicy taste that makes it a popular ingredient in both sweet and savory dishes. In traditional medicine, particularly in Ayurveda and Traditional Chinese Medicine, cinnamon has been prized for its warming nature and its ability to stimulate circulation, enhance digestion, and support the immune system.

In this chapter, we'll explore the medicinal properties of cinnamon, from its powerful anti-inflammatory effects to its role in regulating blood sugar and boosting immunity. Cinnamon's wide range of health benefits makes it a potent spice for natural wellness, easily incorporated into daily meals and beverages.

Medicinal Importance of Cinnamon

Cinnamon is rich in antioxidants, essential oils, and active compounds like cinnamaldehyde, cinnamic acid, and polyphenols, which contribute to its health benefits. Here's how cinnamon can support various aspects of health:

1. Blood Sugar Regulation

Cinnamon is renowned for its ability to help regulate blood sugar levels, making it a valuable spice for those with diabetes or insulin resistance. Compounds in cinnamon improve insulin sensitivity, enabling cells to use glucose more effectively. Studies have shown that cinnamon can help reduce fasting blood sugar levels and improve hemoglobin A1c, a marker of long-term blood sugar control.

- **Blood Sugar Balancing Tip**: Add a pinch of cinnamon powder to your morning oatmeal, smoothies, or coffee to help manage blood sugar levels throughout the day.

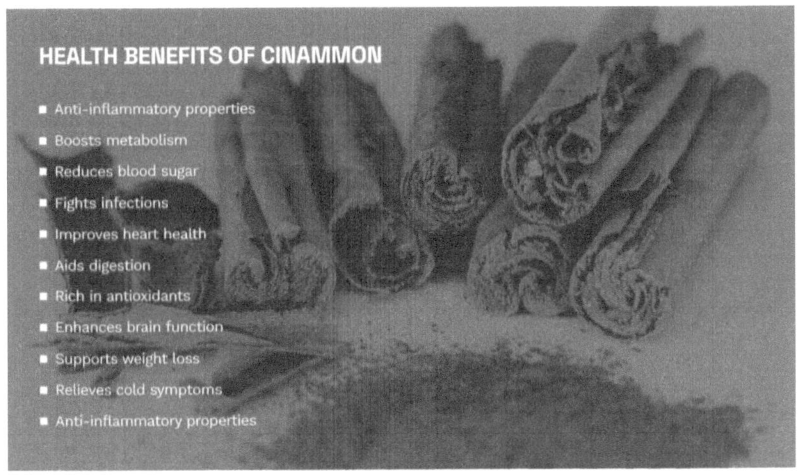

2. Anti-Inflammatory Properties

Cinnamon is rich in anti-inflammatory compounds that can help reduce inflammation in the body. Chronic inflammation is associated with numerous health issues, including heart disease, arthritis, and certain cancers. By reducing inflammatory markers, cinnamon supports overall health and can alleviate symptoms of inflammatory conditions.

- **Anti-Inflammatory Drink**: A warm cup of cinnamon tea can provide soothing relief from inflammation, particularly helpful for individuals with arthritis or joint pain.

3. Antioxidant Powerhouse

Cinnamon is packed with antioxidants like polyphenols, which protect the body from oxidative stress and free radical damage. These antioxidants play a role in reducing the risk of chronic diseases, slowing the aging process, and supporting cellular health. In fact, cinnamon is known to have one of the highest antioxidant contents among spices.

- **Boosting Antioxidant Intake**: Incorporate cinnamon into your diet by sprinkling it over fruits, yogurt, or cereals to enjoy its powerful antioxidant benefits.

4. Supports Heart Health

Cinnamon's heart-protective properties come from its ability to lower LDL (bad) cholesterol and triglycerides while raising HDL (good) cholesterol levels. Additionally, its anti-inflammatory effects reduce the risk of heart disease by decreasing inflammation in blood vessels. Cinnamon may also help regulate blood pressure, contributing further to cardiovascular wellness.

- **Heart-Healthy Tip**: Drinking a cup of cinnamon tea daily or adding a small amount of cinnamon powder to your meals can support heart health.

5. Boosts Immune System

Cinnamon has natural antimicrobial, antibacterial, and antiviral properties, making it effective in fighting infections and strengthening the immune system. This is particularly helpful during cold and flu season. Cinnamon's essential oils can help inhibit the growth of bacteria, fungi, and viruses, promoting overall immune resilience.

- **Immune-Boosting Tea**: Brew cinnamon with ginger and honey in hot water to create a potent immune-boosting drink, especially beneficial for relieving cold and flu symptoms.

6. Improves Digestive Health

Cinnamon is a warming spice that stimulates digestion and helps prevent digestive issues like bloating, indigestion, and nausea. By promoting the secretion of digestive enzymes, cinnamon aids in breaking down food and easing digestion. Its antibacterial properties also help maintain a healthy balance of gut bacteria.

- **Digestive Aid**: Drinking cinnamon tea after a meal or adding cinnamon powder to foods can help reduce bloating and improve digestion.

7. Reduces Risk of Neurodegenerative Diseases

Emerging research suggests that cinnamon may play a role in protecting brain health and reducing the risk of neurodegenerative diseases like Alzheimer's and Parkinson's. Compounds in cinnamon inhibit the buildup of tau proteins, which are associated with Alzheimer's disease, and may improve motor function and cognitive health.

- **Brain Health Support**: Adding cinnamon to daily meals and drinks is an easy way to incorporate its neuroprotective properties into your diet.

8. Relieves Menstrual Cramps and PMS Symptoms

Cinnamon's antispasmodic and anti-inflammatory properties make it a valuable remedy for menstrual cramps and symptoms of premenstrual syndrome (PMS). Cinnamon helps relax muscles, reduce inflammation, and alleviate pain, making it a natural alternative to over-the-counter pain relievers.

- **Menstrual Pain Relief**: Drinking cinnamon tea or sprinkling cinnamon powder into warm milk during menstruation can help relieve cramps and improve comfort.

9. Supports Oral Health

Cinnamon has been used for centuries as a natural remedy for oral health issues. Its antimicrobial properties make it effective in reducing harmful bacteria in the mouth, freshening breath, and preventing gum infections. The essential oils in cinnamon can help combat bad breath and maintain oral hygiene.

- **Oral Health Remedy**: Chewing on a small piece of cinnamon bark or adding cinnamon powder to homemade mouthwash can support oral health.

10. Promotes Healthy Skin

Cinnamon's antimicrobial and antioxidant properties make it beneficial for maintaining healthy, clear skin. It can help treat acne and other skin infections, and its anti-inflammatory effects can reduce redness and irritation. Cinnamon also promotes circulation, which can give the skin a natural glow.

- **Skin-Glow Mask**: Mixing cinnamon powder with honey and applying it as a face mask can help reduce acne and promote a healthy complexion.

Incorporating Cinnamon into Daily Life

Cinnamon can be used in a variety of ways, making it easy to incorporate into your daily routine for health benefits:

- **Cinnamon Tea**: Boil cinnamon sticks in water to make a warm, comforting tea that promotes digestion, boosts immunity, and supports heart health.

- **Cooking**: Add ground cinnamon to a wide range of dishes, from curries to desserts and smoothies. Its flavor enhances both savory and sweet recipes.

- **Cinnamon-Infused Water**: Soak a cinnamon stick in water overnight and drink it throughout the day for mild, steady health benefits, including blood sugar regulation.

Ayurvedic Context of Cinnamon

Cinnamon (*Cinnamomum verum*), known as *Tvak* in Sanskrit, is one of Ayurveda's most revered spices. Often referred to as the "sweet healer," cinnamon has been used for centuries for its warming, stimulating, and rejuvenating properties. In Ayurveda, it is valued not only as a flavorful spice but also as a potent medicinal herb with a range of health benefits for the body and mind.

Dosha Balancing Properties

Cinnamon is primarily known for its ability to balance *Vata* and *Kapha* doshas due to its heating (*ushna*) nature, light (*laghu*) quality, and sweet (*madhura*) and pungent (*katu*) taste. It stimulates warmth, circulation, and metabolic activity, making it an excellent remedy for cold and sluggish conditions associated with *Vata* and *Kapha* imbalances.

While cinnamon's warming properties may mildly aggravate *Pitta* when consumed in excess, its sweet taste helps to moderate this effect, allowing it to be used sparingly even by individuals with *Pitta* dominance.

Digestive and Metabolic Support

In Ayurveda, cinnamon is highly valued for its digestive properties (*deepana* and *pachana*), which help to stimulate the digestive fire (*Agni*) and enhance the assimilation of nutrients. It is particularly effective in alleviating symptoms of indigestion, bloating, and gas. A pinch of cinnamon powder added to warm water or herbal teas can promote digestive comfort and prevent sluggish digestion.

Cinnamon is also known for its ability to regulate blood sugar levels and improve insulin sensitivity, making it a key herb in Ayurvedic treatments for diabetes and metabolic disorders. Its thermogenic properties help to boost metabolism and aid in weight management by reducing cravings and balancing blood sugar.

Circulatory and Cardiovascular Health

Cinnamon is a powerful circulatory stimulant (*Vyana Vayu*), which promotes healthy blood flow and supports cardiovascular health. It helps to lower cholesterol levels, reduce blood pressure, and improve overall heart function. In Ayurveda, cinnamon is often used in formulations to enhance circulation, warm the body, and alleviate cold hands and feet.

Anti-Inflammatory and Immune-Boosting Properties

Cinnamon's anti-inflammatory and antimicrobial properties make it a valuable herb for boosting immunity and fighting infections. It is often used to alleviate respiratory conditions such as colds, coughs, and bronchitis by clearing mucus, reducing congestion, and soothing sore throats. A traditional Ayurvedic remedy involves boiling cinnamon sticks with ginger and honey to create a warming, immune-boosting tea.

Rejuvenation and Detoxification

Cinnamon is considered a mild rejuvenative (*Rasayana*) in Ayurveda, promoting vitality, mental clarity, and overall well-being. Its detoxifying properties help to eliminate toxins (*ama*) from the body, purify the blood, and support healthy liver function.

In Ayurveda, cinnamon is more than just a spice—it is a holistic healer that supports digestion, circulation, and immunity, making it a vital component of a balanced, health-conscious lifestyle.

Precautions

While cinnamon is generally safe, it is best to consume it in moderation. Cassia cinnamon, the most common type, contains coumarin, a compound that can be harmful in large quantities and may affect liver health. Opting for Ceylon cinnamon, which has lower levels of coumarin, can help reduce this risk. Individuals taking blood-thinning medications or those with liver issues should consult a healthcare provider before consuming cinnamon supplements or in large amounts.

Conclusion

Cinnamon's medicinal benefits make it an essential spice in the kitchen and an invaluable part of natural medicine. From supporting heart health and blood sugar balance to boosting immunity and reducing inflammation, cinnamon has a wide range of healing properties that can enhance daily wellness. Its unique flavor and versatility in both culinary and medicinal applications have kept it popular for centuries. By incorporating cinnamon into meals and home remedies, you can enjoy the potent benefits of this warming healer, adding a touch of spice to both your diet and your health routine.

<u>RECIPES</u>

Cinnamon (Cinnamomum spp.) is a versatile spice with powerful medicinal properties. It is known for its anti-inflammatory, antimicrobial, and blood sugar-lowering effects. Below are some effective medicinal recipes using cinnamon:

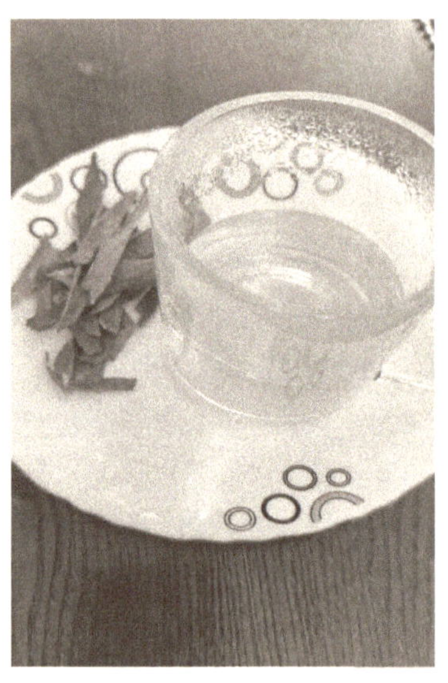

1. Cinnamon Tea for Digestion and Immunity

Improves digestion, boosts immunity, and soothes sore throats.

Ingredients:

- 1 stick of cinnamon (or 1 teaspoon cinnamon powder)
- 1 cup water
- Honey (optional)

Instructions:

1. Boil the water and add the cinnamon stick or powder.
2. Simmer for 10 minutes and strain.
3. Add honey if desired, and drink warm.

2. Cinnamon and Honey Paste for Cough and Sore Throat

Relieves cough, soothes the throat, and fights infections.
Ingredients:

- 1 teaspoon cinnamon powder

- 1 tablespoon honey

Instructions:

1. Mix cinnamon powder with honey into a smooth paste.

2. Take 1 teaspoon twice daily until symptoms improve.

3. Cinnamon Water for Blood Sugar Control

Helps regulate blood sugar levels and boosts metabolism.
Ingredients:

- 1 stick of cinnamon

- 1 cup water

Instructions:

1. Soak the cinnamon stick in water overnight.

2. Drink the infused water on an empty stomach in the morning.

4. Cinnamon and Turmeric Milk for Inflammation

Reduces inflammation and promotes better sleep.

Ingredients:

- 1/2 teaspoon cinnamon powder
- 1/4 teaspoon turmeric powder
- 1 cup milk
- Honey (optional)

Instructions:

1. Heat the milk and add cinnamon and turmeric.
2. Stir well and simmer for 5 minutes.
3. Sweeten with honey if desired, and drink warm.

5. Cinnamon Oil for Joint Pain Relief

Soothes aching joints and reduces inflammation.

Ingredients:

- 2 tablespoons cinnamon powder
- 1/2 cup coconut or olive oil

Instructions:

1. Heat the oil and add cinnamon powder.
2. Let it simmer for 10 minutes, then strain.
3. Massage onto affected areas as needed.

6. Cinnamon Face Mask for Glowing Skin

Brightens skin and helps fight acne.
Ingredients:

- 1 teaspoon cinnamon powder

- 2 tablespoons honey

Instructions:

1. Mix cinnamon powder and honey into a paste.

2. Apply to the face and leave on for 10-15 minutes.

3. Rinse with warm water. Use once a week.

7. Cinnamon Detox Drink for Weight Loss

Boosts metabolism and aids fat loss.
Ingredients:

- 1 stick of cinnamon

- Juice of half a lemon

- 1 cup warm water

Instructions:

1. Add the cinnamon stick to warm water and let it steep for 5-10 minutes.

2. Add lemon juice and stir.

3. Drink on an empty stomach daily.

---

8. Cinnamon and Ginger Tea for Cold Relief

Alleviates cold symptoms, clears sinuses, and boosts immunity.
Ingredients:

- 1 stick of cinnamon

- 1-inch piece of ginger, sliced

- 1 cup water

- Honey (optional)

Instructions:

1. Boil water with cinnamon and ginger slices for 10 minutes.

2. Strain and sweeten with honey if desired.

3. Drink warm during cold symptoms.

---

9. Cinnamon Powder for Bad Breath

Freshens breath and kills bacteria in the mouth.
Ingredients:

- 1/2 teaspoon cinnamon powder

- 1 cup warm water

Instructions:

1. Mix cinnamon powder in warm water.

2. Use as a mouth rinse after brushing teeth.

10. Cinnamon Infused Honey for Heart Health

Lowers cholesterol, improves heart health, and boosts energy.
Ingredients:

- 2 tablespoons honey

- 1 teaspoon cinnamon powder

Instructions:

1. Mix honey and cinnamon into a smooth paste.

2. Take 1 teaspoon daily, preferably in the morning.

These recipes demonstrate the diverse medicinal uses of cinnamon for health and wellness. Always consult a healthcare provider before using cinnamon as a remedy if you have specific medical conditions or take medications.

Common Myths and Misconceptions About Cinnamon

Cinnamon, often hailed as a "super spice," has been treasured for its aroma, flavor, and health benefits. However, its widespread use has also led to the emergence of myths and misconceptions. Let's separate fact from fiction when it comes to cinnamon.

1. All Types of Cinnamon Are the Same

Myth: All cinnamon varieties offer identical taste and health benefits.

Reality: There are two primary types of cinnamon: **Ceylon cinnamon** (true cinnamon) and **Cassia cinnamon**. Ceylon is considered the "true" cinnamon with a milder flavor and lower levels of coumarin, making it safer for long-term use. Cassia is more common and affordable but contains higher levels of coumarin, which can be harmful in excessive amounts.

2. Cinnamon Can Cure Diabetes

Myth: Cinnamon is a standalone cure for diabetes.

Reality: Cinnamon can help lower blood sugar levels and improve insulin sensitivity, but it is not a cure. It should be used as part of a comprehensive diabetes management plan that includes a balanced diet, exercise, and medication if needed.

3. Eating More Cinnamon Is Always Better

Myth: The more cinnamon you consume, the greater the health benefits.

Reality: Excessive consumption, especially of Cassia cinnamon, can lead to health risks such as liver damage due to high coumarin content. Stick to moderate amounts—about 1 to 2 teaspoons per day for most people.

4. Cinnamon Has No Side Effects

Myth: Cinnamon is completely safe for everyone.

Reality: While generally safe in culinary amounts, excessive intake can cause side effects like mouth irritation, low blood sugar, or allergic reactions. Cassia cinnamon in high doses poses a risk of liver toxicity.

5. Cinnamon Helps Everyone Lose Weight Instantly

Myth: Cinnamon is a miracle spice for quick and easy weight loss.

Reality: Cinnamon may support weight management by boosting metabolism and controlling blood sugar levels, but it is not a magic solution. Sustainable weight loss requires a healthy lifestyle, not just a sprinkle of cinnamon.

6. Cinnamon Is Only Useful as a Spice

Myth: Cinnamon is only good for cooking and flavoring food.
Reality: Cinnamon has medicinal and cosmetic applications too. It can be used as an anti-inflammatory agent, for improving circulation, and even in skincare to reduce acne or brighten skin.

7. Cinnamon Tea Alone Can Prevent Colds and Flu

Myth: Drinking cinnamon tea daily will completely protect you from getting sick.
Reality: Cinnamon has antimicrobial and warming properties that can support immunity and soothe cold symptoms, but it's not a guaranteed shield against infections. Pair it with a healthy diet and proper hygiene for better protection.

8. Cinnamon Powder Is Always Pure

Myth: Cinnamon powder available in stores is always pure and authentic.
Reality: Ground cinnamon is often mixed with fillers or low-quality varieties. To ensure authenticity, buy from reputable sources or grind your cinnamon sticks at home.

9. Cinnamon Can Be Stored Indefinitely

Myth: Cinnamon doesn't spoil and can be stored forever without losing potency.

Reality: While cinnamon has a long shelf life, it loses its flavor and medicinal potency over time. Ground cinnamon typically lasts about six months to a year, while cinnamon sticks can last 2–3 years when stored in an airtight container.

10. Cinnamon Can Be Safely Taken in Any Condition

Myth: Cinnamon is universally safe and can be consumed in any health condition.

Reality: People on blood-thinning medications, those with liver disease, or individuals prone to hypoglycemia should be cautious with cinnamon, especially Cassia. Consult a healthcare provider if in doubt.

By debunking these myths, we can better appreciate cinnamon's true power and versatility. This warm and aromatic spice, when used correctly, is a delightful addition to both your kitchen and your wellness routine.

Chapter 7: Cloves – The Powerful Antiseptic

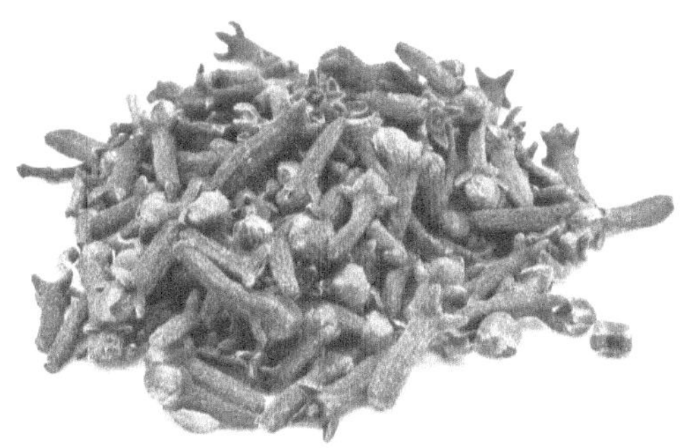

Introduction

Cloves, known as *Laung* in Hindi, are aromatic flower buds from the *Syzygium aromaticum* tree and have been valued for centuries in both culinary and medicinal traditions. With a distinct warm, sweet-spicy aroma, cloves are commonly used to flavor food, but their medicinal uses are equally notable. Packed with beneficial compounds such as eugenol, cloves have been used in traditional medicine as an antiseptic, analgesic, and digestive aid. Their potent antioxidant and anti-inflammatory properties make them an invaluable spice for promoting overall health and well-being.

In this chapter, we'll delve into the medicinal uses of cloves, from their ability to relieve pain and improve digestion to their role in enhancing immunity. Cloves are small but powerful, offering a range of natural benefits that make them an essential addition to the kitchen and home remedies.

Medicinal Importance of Cloves

Cloves are rich in essential oils, antioxidants, vitamins, and minerals, contributing to their extensive health benefits. Here's how cloves can support health and address common ailments:

1. Natural Pain Reliever

Cloves contain eugenol, a compound with natural analgesic properties that can provide effective pain relief. This makes cloves particularly helpful for relieving toothaches, sore gums, and headaches. Eugenol works as a mild anaesthetic, numbing the area where it's applied and providing temporary relief from pain.

- **Toothache Relief**: Applying a drop of clove oil or placing a whole clove near the aching tooth can help alleviate pain until professional dental care is available.

2. Powerful Antiseptic and Antibacterial

Cloves are known for their antiseptic and antibacterial properties, which make them effective in combating bacterial infections and preventing infections in minor wounds or cuts. The eugenol in cloves acts as a natural antimicrobial, inhibiting the growth of harmful bacteria and reducing the risk of infections.

- **Antibacterial Mouth Rinse**: Clove-infused water can be used as a natural mouthwash to kill oral bacteria, freshen breath, and maintain oral hygiene.

3. Supports Digestive Health

Cloves are commonly used in traditional remedies to aid digestion. They stimulate the production of digestive enzymes, reduce bloating, and alleviate gas. Cloves can also help soothe stomach discomfort and reduce nausea, making them beneficial for people who experience digestive issues frequently.

- **Digestive Aid**: Drinking warm water infused with a few cloves or adding ground cloves to meals can ease bloating, indigestion, and other digestive discomforts.

HEALTH BENEFITS OF CLOVES

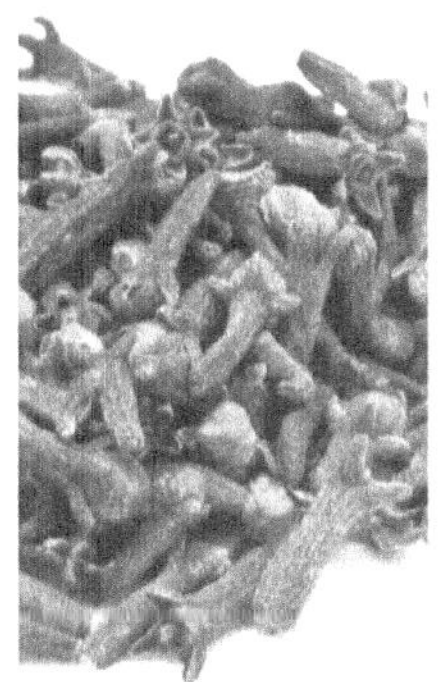

4. Anti-Inflammatory Benefits

The anti-inflammatory properties of cloves, largely due to eugenol, help reduce inflammation in the body. Cloves can be used to relieve inflammation associated with conditions such as arthritis, joint pain, and skin irritation. They also help lower inflammatory markers, which may reduce the risk of chronic diseases linked to inflammation.

- **Joint Pain Remedy**: Applying diluted clove oil to sore joints or muscles can provide relief from inflammation and reduce pain.

5. Rich in Antioxidants

Cloves are packed with antioxidants, particularly phenolic compounds, which help neutralize free radicals in the body. These antioxidants help protect cells from oxidative stress, which is linked to aging and the development of chronic diseases. Regular consumption of cloves may support cellular health and reduce the risk of cancer and heart disease.

- **Antioxidant Boost**: Adding cloves to daily meals or drinking clove tea can increase antioxidant intake and support overall health.

6. Immune System Booster

Cloves are natural immune boosters, thanks to their antibacterial, antiviral, and antifungal properties. They help the body fight infections and support the immune system in staying resilient, particularly during cold and flu season. Cloves can help prevent respiratory infections and ease symptoms of colds and coughs.

- **Immunity-Boosting Drink**: Adding cloves to warm tea with honey and ginger is a great way to strengthen immunity and soothe respiratory discomforts.

7. Improves Respiratory Health

Cloves can be helpful in managing respiratory ailments like asthma, bronchitis, and coughs. The essential oils in cloves help loosen mucus and reduce throat irritation, making them effective for relieving respiratory symptoms. Clove's antimicrobial properties also help fight respiratory infections, providing relief from congestion and cough.

- **Cough Remedy**: Sipping clove-infused tea or chewing on a clove can relieve coughs and soothe sore throats, making it easier to breathe and reducing irritation.

8. Enhances Oral Health

Cloves are a traditional remedy for oral health due to their antiseptic and analgesic properties. They help relieve toothaches, fight bacteria in the mouth, and prevent bad breath. Clove oil is often used in dental treatments for its ability to numb pain and kill bacteria, making it an effective ingredient for oral care.

- **Natural Mouth Freshener**: Chewing on a clove after meals can help eliminate bad breath and support oral hygiene by killing harmful bacteria.

9. Supports Liver Health

Eugenol in cloves has been shown to help promote liver health by reducing inflammation and oxidative stress in the liver. It may also protect the liver from damage caused by toxins and support overall liver function, which is essential for detoxification and digestion.

- **Liver Health Tip**: Including cloves in the diet in moderation can support liver health, especially when combined with other liver-supporting spices like turmeric.

10. Potential Anti-Cancer Properties

Some studies suggest that cloves may have anti-cancer properties due to their high antioxidant content and the presence of eugenol, which has shown potential in inhibiting the growth of certain cancer cells. While more research is needed, cloves are believed to reduce the risk of cancer by fighting free radicals and protecting cellular health.

- **Daily Antioxidant Routine**: Adding cloves to meals or using clove oil in moderation may help contribute to a diet rich in cancer-fighting antioxidants.

Incorporating Cloves into Daily Life

Cloves are versatile and can be used in various ways, from cooking to home remedies:

- **Clove Tea**: Boil a few cloves in water to make a warm, spicy tea that soothes the throat, aids digestion, and supports immunity.

- **Cooking**: Add cloves to curries, soups, stews, and spiced drinks. They pair well with both sweet and savory dishes.

- **Clove Oil**: Dilute clove oil with a carrier oil for topical applications, such as for joint pain, sore gums, or skin issues.

Ayurvedic Context of Cloves

Cloves (*Syzygium aromaticum*), known as *Laung* in Sanskrit, are one of the most powerful and widely used spices in Ayurveda. Revered for their pungent taste, warming properties, and numerous therapeutic benefits, cloves have been utilized for thousands of years to promote overall health and wellness. In Ayurveda, cloves are considered a *Vishwabhesaj* (universal medicine), meaning they can treat a wide range of ailments and balance the body's energies.

Dosha Balancing Properties

Cloves are known for their ability to balance *Vata* and *Kapha* doshas due to their warming (*ushna*) and stimulating qualities. They are rich in pungent (*katu*) and bitter (*tikta*) flavors, which make them effective for alleviating excess cold, dampness, and stagnation in the body. This is particularly helpful in cases of digestive sluggishness, poor circulation, and respiratory congestion caused by *Kapha* imbalances.

However, due to their heating nature, cloves can mildly aggravate *Pitta* dosha, especially in individuals with a *Pitta*-dominant constitution or during hot weather. As such, cloves should be used in moderation to avoid excess heat in the body.

Digestive and Metabolic Support

In Ayurveda, cloves are highly valued for their ability to stimulate the digestive fire (*Agni*), improving digestion, absorption, and elimination. Cloves are known to relieve nausea, indigestion, bloating, and flatulence by promoting the secretion of digestive enzymes. A common Ayurvedic remedy involves boiling a few cloves in water and drinking the decoction to soothe stomach discomfort and improve appetite.

Cloves also aid in balancing the metabolic process by enhancing circulation, increasing body temperature, and promoting better digestion. They are often included in detoxification and weight loss regimens due to their ability to help burn toxins (*ama*) and support the body's natural cleansing mechanisms.

Anti-Inflammatory and Pain Relief

Cloves possess powerful anti-inflammatory and analgesic properties. They are used in Ayurveda to alleviate pain, reduce swelling, and manage conditions such as arthritis, joint pain, and muscle stiffness. Clove oil is often massaged onto sore muscles and joints for its local pain-relieving effect. Internally, cloves help reduce inflammation in the gastrointestinal tract, which can be beneficial in managing conditions like ulcers and gastritis.

Respiratory and Immune Support

Cloves are renowned for their ability to relieve respiratory issues, such as cough, cold, sore throat, and bronchitis. Their antiseptic and expectorant properties help clear mucus, soothe irritated airways, and relieve congestion. A decoction of cloves, ginger, and honey is a traditional Ayurvedic remedy for respiratory discomfort.

Additionally, cloves are rich in antioxidants and possess strong antimicrobial properties, which support immune health and help fight infections. Regular use of cloves can enhance the body's natural defense mechanisms, making it effective in boosting overall immunity.

Detoxification and Oral Health

In Ayurveda, cloves are used for detoxifying the body by purging toxins from the digestive tract and supporting the liver. Their anti-toxic properties promote liver health and help purify the blood.

Cloves also have significant benefits for oral health. They are used to treat toothaches, gums infections, and bad breath due to their antimicrobial and analgesic properties. A clove-infused mouthwash or clove oil can soothe dental discomfort and kill bacteria in the mouth, promoting better oral hygiene.

In summary, cloves are a versatile and potent herb in Ayurveda, used to balance the doshas, stimulate digestion, relieve pain and inflammation, support respiratory health, and boost immunity. Their wide array of benefits makes them an essential spice in the Ayurvedic approach to health and healing.

Precautions

Cloves are potent, so it's important to use them in moderation. Excessive consumption of cloves or clove oil can cause digestive discomfort and may irritate sensitive skin. Additionally, clove oil should be diluted before topical use to avoid skin irritation. Pregnant or breastfeeding women and individuals on anticoagulant medications should consult a healthcare provider before using cloves medicinally.

Conclusion

Cloves are a small but powerful spice that packs a wealth of health benefits. From relieving pain and enhancing digestive health to boosting immunity and supporting liver function, cloves play a vital role in natural medicine. Their antibacterial, anti-inflammatory, and antioxidant properties make them a valuable addition to daily wellness routines. By incorporating cloves into meals, beverages, and remedies, you can enjoy the multitude of healing benefits this spice has to offer. As a kitchen staple and a natural healer, cloves embody the enduring power of nature's remedies.

<u>RECIPES</u>

Here are **10 medicinal recipes featuring cloves**, a potent spice known for its antimicrobial, anti-inflammatory, and pain-relieving properties. Cloves are widely used in traditional

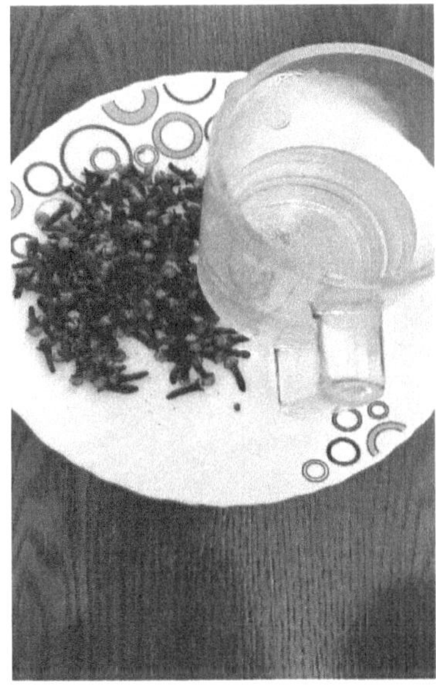

1. Clove Tea for Digestion

A soothing drink to alleviate bloating and indigestion.

Ingredients:

- 3–4 cloves

- 1 cup water

- 1 teaspoon honey (optional)

Instructions:

1. Boil water and add cloves.

2. Simmer for 5 minutes, strain, and sweeten with honey if desired.

Benefits: Improves digestion, reduces bloating, and soothes stomach discomfort.

2. Clove Gargle for Sore Throat

A natural remedy for throat irritation and infections.

Ingredients:

- 4 cloves
- 1 cup boiling water
- A pinch of salt

Instructions:

1. Steep cloves in boiling water for 10 minutes.
2. Add salt and gargle with the solution.

Benefits: Relieves sore throat, kills bacteria, and soothes inflammation.

---

3. Clove and Honey Remedy for Cough

A quick remedy to ease coughs and congestion.

Ingredients:

- 1 teaspoon clove powder
- 1 teaspoon honey

Instructions:

1. Mix clove powder with honey.
2. Consume 1 teaspoon 2–3 times a day.

Benefits: Reduces cough, clears mucus, and fights respiratory infections.

4. Clove Oil for Toothache Relief

A classic solution for dental pain and gum health.

Ingredients:

- 2–3 drops clove oil
- Cotton ball

Instructions:

1. Dab clove oil onto the cotton ball.
2. Apply directly to the affected tooth or gum area.

Benefits: Relieves toothache, reduces gum inflammation, and fights bacteria.

5. Clove and Ginger Detox Tea

A warming drink for detoxification and immunity.

Ingredients:

- 4 cloves
- 1-inch piece of fresh ginger (grated)
- 1 cup water
- Juice of 1/2 lemon

Instructions:

1. Boil water with cloves and ginger for 5 minutes.

2. Strain, add lemon juice, and serve warm.

Benefits: Boosts metabolism, aids detoxification, and improves digestion.

---

6. Clove Steam Inhalation for Congestion

A simple therapy to clear sinuses and respiratory passages.

Ingredients:

- 5 cloves

- 4 cups boiling water

Instructions:

1. Add cloves to boiling water.

2. Inhale the steam under a towel for 5–10 minutes.

Benefits: Clears nasal congestion, relieves sinus pressure, and soothes respiratory discomfort.

---

7. Clove Milk for Better Sleep

A comforting drink to promote relaxation and fight insomnia.

Ingredients:

- 1 cup warm milk

- 2–3 cloves

- 1 teaspoon honey

Instructions:

1. Heat milk and add cloves.

2. Simmer for 5 minutes, strain, and sweeten with honey.

Benefits: Reduces stress, improves sleep quality, and eases muscle tension.

8. Clove Face Pack for Acne

A natural remedy for clear, blemish-free skin.

Ingredients:

- 1 teaspoon clove powder

- 1 tablespoon honey

- 1 tablespoon yogurt

Instructions:

1. Mix all ingredients into a paste.

2. Apply to the face and leave for 10–15 minutes.

3. Rinse with lukewarm water.

Benefits: Fights acne-causing bacteria, reduces inflammation, and brightens skin.

9. Clove Water for Immunity

A simple tonic to strengthen your immune system.

Ingredients:

- 5 cloves
- 2 cups water

Instructions:

1. Boil water with cloves for 10 minutes.
2. Strain and sip throughout the day.

Benefits: Enhances immunity, fights infections, and provides antioxidants.

---

10. Clove and Cinnamon Herbal Infusion

A warming drink for cold relief and energy.

Ingredients:

- 4 cloves
- 1 small cinnamon stick
- 1 cup water
- 1 teaspoon honey

Instructions:

1. Boil water with cloves and cinnamon for 5 minutes.
2. Strain, sweeten with honey, and serve warm.

Benefits: Relieves cold symptoms, boosts energy, and soothes inflammation.

These clove-based medicinal recipes are easy to prepare and offer natural solutions for common health concerns. Incorporate them into your daily routine to experience the healing power of cloves!

Common Myths and Misconceptions About Cloves

Cloves, the aromatic flower buds used in cuisines and remedies worldwide, are prized for their medicinal and culinary properties. However, they are also surrounded by myths and misconceptions that often lead to misuse or undervaluation. Let's set the record straight on this powerful spice.

1. Cloves Are Just a Flavoring Agent

Myth: Cloves are only useful for enhancing the taste of food and drinks.

Reality: While cloves add a distinct flavor to dishes, they are also packed with medicinal properties. Cloves have antimicrobial, anti-inflammatory, and antioxidant effects, making them valuable for health beyond their culinary uses.

2. Clove Oil Can Be Applied Directly to Any Skin Problem

Myth: Clove oil is safe for direct application to treat any skin issue.

Reality: Clove oil is potent and can irritate the skin if applied undiluted. It should always be diluted with a carrier oil before use and tested on a small area first.

3. Cloves Cure Toothaches Permanently

Myth: A clove or clove oil can completely cure toothaches and dental problems.

Reality: Cloves provide temporary relief from tooth pain due to their natural anesthetic and antibacterial properties. However, they do not address the underlying cause of dental issues, which requires professional treatment.

4. Cloves Are Unsafe During Pregnancy

Myth: Consuming cloves during pregnancy can harm the mother or baby.

Reality: Cloves are generally safe in culinary amounts during pregnancy. However, clove oil or supplements should only be used under medical supervision, as their high potency may pose risks.

5. Cloves Can Be Consumed in Unlimited Quantities

Myth: Eating large quantities of cloves increases their health benefits.

Reality: Overconsumption of cloves can lead to adverse effects like digestive discomfort, low blood sugar, or an increased risk of bleeding due to their blood-thinning properties. Moderation is key.

6. Cloves Are Effective Against All Types of Infections

Myth: Cloves are a universal remedy for any infection.
Reality: Cloves have antimicrobial properties and can help combat certain bacteria and fungi, but they are not effective against all infections. They should complement, not replace, appropriate medical treatments.

7. Cloves Are Only Used in Indian Cuisine

Myth: Cloves are exclusively used in Indian dishes like biryanis and curries.
Reality: Cloves are a global spice, used in Middle Eastern, African, and Western cuisines. They are a key ingredient in spice blends like Chinese five-spice and garam masala, as well as in beverages like mulled wine and chai.

8. Cloves Are Only Medicinal When Used Whole

Myth: Only whole cloves retain medicinal benefits, and ground cloves are ineffective.
Reality: Ground cloves retain most of their medicinal properties if stored properly, though they lose potency faster than whole cloves. Both forms can provide health benefits when used correctly.

9. Cloves Are a Cure-All for Respiratory Issues

Myth: Cloves can completely cure respiratory problems like asthma or bronchitis.

Reality: Cloves can help ease symptoms like congestion and cough due to their anti-inflammatory and expectorant properties, but they are not a standalone cure. Medical intervention is essential for chronic or severe conditions.

10. Cloves Are Harmless for Everyone

Myth: Cloves have no side effects and can be consumed by anyone.

Reality: Cloves may interact with certain medications, particularly blood thinners, and can cause allergic reactions or digestive discomfort in some individuals. Always consult a healthcare provider if unsure about using cloves medicinally.

By busting these myths, we can better understand and use cloves for their true potential. This small yet mighty spice deserves respect for its remarkable flavor and health benefits when used wisely.

Chapter 8: Black Pepper – The King of Spices

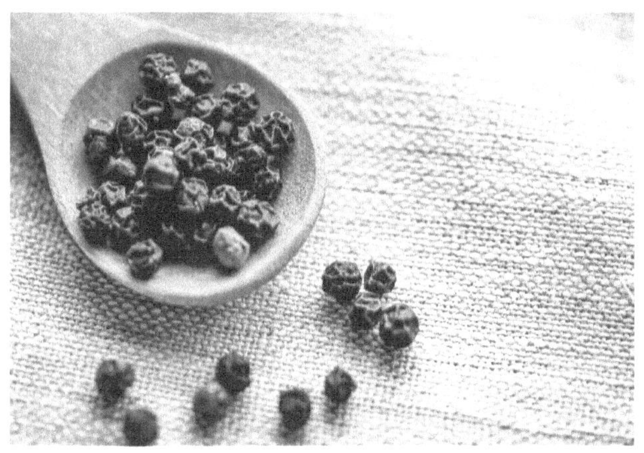

Introduction

Black pepper, often referred to as the "King of Spices," is one of the oldest and most widely used spices in the world. Known as *Kali Mirch* in Hindi, black pepper is derived from the dried fruit of the *Piper nigrum* plant. This versatile spice is celebrated not only for its pungent, sharp flavor but also for its extensive medicinal properties. In traditional medicine systems like Ayurveda and Traditional Chinese Medicine, black pepper has been used as a powerful remedy for various ailments, from digestive issues to respiratory conditions.

In this chapter, we will explore the numerous medicinal benefits of black pepper, from its role in enhancing digestion and boosting metabolism to its ability to act as a natural detoxifier and immune booster. Its active compound, piperine, is responsible for many of its health-promoting effects and makes black pepper a valuable addition to daily meals and home remedies.

Medicinal Importance of Black Pepper

Black pepper is rich in essential oils, antioxidants, and vitamins, which collectively contribute to its therapeutic effects. Here's how black pepper can promote health and aid in the treatment of various conditions:

1. Enhances Digestive Health

Black pepper stimulates the production of digestive enzymes, making it highly beneficial for digestion. Piperine, its active compound, improves the bioavailability of nutrients and other compounds, helping the body absorb them more efficiently. Black pepper can alleviate indigestion, reduce bloating, and prevent constipation.

- **Digestive Aid**: Adding a pinch of black pepper to meals can stimulate digestive juices and improve the absorption of nutrients, reducing the risk of digestive discomfort.

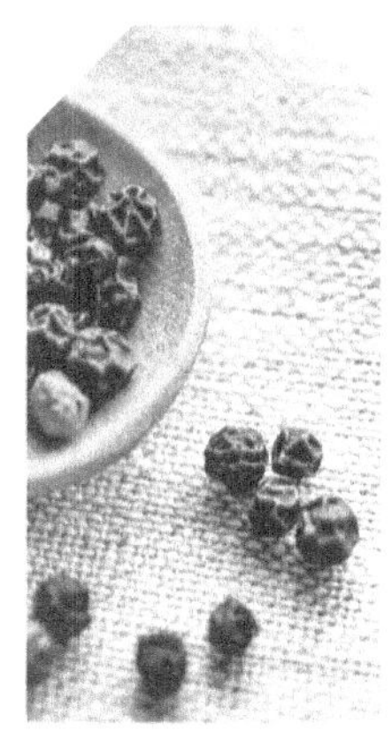

2. Boosts Metabolism and Aids Weight Loss

Black pepper is a natural thermogenic agent, meaning it can increase body heat and help boost metabolism. This thermogenic effect helps the body burn more calories, making black pepper a useful spice for those aiming to lose weight or manage their body composition. Additionally, piperine may inhibit the formation of new fat cells.

- **Weight Loss Tip**: A pinch of black pepper in a glass of warm water with lemon can be consumed in the morning to jump-start metabolism and aid in weight loss.

3. Rich in Antioxidants

Black pepper is a rich source of antioxidants that protect the body from free radical damage, which is linked to aging and chronic diseases like cancer and heart disease. Piperine enhances the antioxidant effects, reducing oxidative stress and promoting cellular health.

- **Antioxidant Boost**: Sprinkle black pepper over fresh fruits, vegetables, or in green smoothies to increase the antioxidant intake and support cellular health.

4. Improves Respiratory Health

Black pepper's warming nature makes it an excellent remedy for respiratory ailments, including coughs, colds, and sinus congestion. It acts as an expectorant, helping to loosen phlegm and clear the respiratory passages. Black pepper's antibacterial properties also help in fighting infections that cause respiratory discomfort.

- **Cold Relief**: Drinking a warm concoction of black pepper, honey, and ginger can soothe a sore throat, relieve coughs, and promote easier breathing.

5. Enhances Nutrient Absorption

One of black pepper's most valuable medicinal properties is its ability to improve the bioavailability of other nutrients and compounds, including curcumin (found in turmeric) and certain vitamins and minerals. Piperine enhances the absorption of these compounds, making it beneficial when used with other spices and supplements.

- **Enhanced Absorption**: Adding black pepper to dishes with turmeric, like golden milk or curries, boosts the absorption of curcumin, maximizing its anti-inflammatory benefits.

6. Anti-Inflammatory Properties

Black pepper contains compounds with anti-inflammatory properties, which help reduce inflammation throughout the body. Chronic inflammation is a risk factor for several diseases, including arthritis, diabetes, and heart disease. Piperine in black pepper helps to inhibit inflammatory markers, making it beneficial for individuals dealing with inflammatory conditions.

- **Joint Health**: Consuming black pepper in meals or as part of herbal teas can help reduce joint pain and inflammation.

7. Supports Immune System

Black pepper's antibacterial and immune-boosting properties make it an effective natural remedy for strengthening the immune system. Its warming nature helps prevent infections and supports the body's defense mechanisms, especially useful during cold and flu season.

- **Immunity Boost**: Adding black pepper to herbal teas or warm broths can support the immune system and help the body fight off infections.

8. Promotes Mental Clarity and Cognitive Health

Research suggests that black pepper may have cognitive-enhancing effects due to its antioxidant properties and its ability to reduce oxidative stress in the brain. Piperine has been shown to improve cognitive function and may protect against neurodegenerative diseases like Alzheimer's and Parkinson's by supporting healthy brain function.

- **Brain Health Tip**: Incorporate black pepper into daily meals to enjoy its neuroprotective effects, especially beneficial as part of a balanced diet for cognitive health.

9. Natural Detoxifier

Black pepper acts as a natural detoxifier by stimulating sweating and urination, which help the body eliminate toxins. Its diaphoretic and diuretic properties assist the liver in flushing out impurities and toxins, promoting a healthier internal system.

- **Detox Drink**: A warm drink with black pepper, lemon, and honey can help cleanse the system, boost metabolism, and support the liver.

10. Potential Anti-Cancer Properties

Some studies suggest that black pepper may have anti-cancer properties, as piperine may slow the growth of cancer cells and inhibit the formation of tumors. Combined with its antioxidant properties, black pepper's effects on cellular health and protection from free radicals may contribute to a reduced risk of cancer.

- **Daily Antioxidant Intake**: Regularly adding black pepper to meals and pairing it with other antioxidant-rich foods may help support long-term cellular health and reduce cancer risk.

Incorporating Black Pepper into Daily Life

Black pepper is versatile and easy to incorporate into daily routines:

- **Cooking**: Add black pepper to a variety of dishes, from curries and soups to salads and eggs, for both flavor and health benefits.

- **Herbal Tea**: Boil black pepper with ginger and honey to make a soothing tea that supports digestion, immunity, and respiratory health.

- **Golden Milk**: Add black pepper to turmeric milk to boost curcumin absorption, enhancing anti-inflammatory and antioxidant effects.

Ayurvedic Context of Black Pepper

Black pepper (*Piper nigrum*), known as *Maricha* in Sanskrit, is one of the most celebrated and potent spices in Ayurveda. Often referred to as the "king of spices," black pepper has been prized for its ability to stimulate digestion, enhance metabolism, and provide therapeutic benefits across a wide range of conditions. In Ayurvedic medicine, it is considered a powerful herb with warming, stimulating, and detoxifying properties.

Dosha Balancing Properties

Black pepper is predominantly used to balance *Vata* and *Kapha* doshas due to its heating (*ushna*) nature and pungent (*katu*) taste. Its stimulating qualities help counterbalance the cold, damp, and sluggish qualities of *Vata* and *Kapha*. It aids in promoting circulation, digestion, and metabolic activity. By enhancing *Agni* (digestive fire), black pepper increases warmth in the body, making it especially beneficial for individuals experiencing digestive stagnation, lethargy, or a tendency toward coldness.

Although black pepper is less likely to aggravate *Pitta*, it should still be used in moderation for individuals with *Pitta*-dominant constitutions, as it can potentially increase heat in the body when consumed in excess.

Digestive and Metabolic Support

In Ayurveda, black pepper is revered for its potent ability to stimulate the digestive fire (*Agni*) and enhance the digestion and absorption of food. It is known to promote better metabolism and alleviate digestive discomfort such as bloating, indigestion, and gas. Black pepper's main active compound, piperine, enhances the bioavailability of other nutrients and compounds in food, ensuring that the body absorbs essential vitamins and minerals efficiently.

Black pepper is also used to support weight management and boost metabolic function. By stimulating circulation and thermogenesis, it helps increase caloric burning and detoxification, making it an effective herb for promoting healthy weight and energy levels.

Respiratory and Immune Support

Black pepper's ability to stimulate the respiratory system and clear nasal passages makes it a valuable herb in treating respiratory ailments. It helps to alleviate symptoms of cough, cold, and bronchitis by loosening mucus and clearing congestion. A common Ayurvedic remedy for cough involves mixing black pepper powder with honey and consuming it to reduce inflammation and soothe the throat.

Additionally, black pepper has antibacterial and antioxidant properties that strengthen the immune system. Its warming effect helps to fight infections and boost the body's natural defenses.

Detoxification and Anti-Inflammatory Properties

Black pepper's natural detoxifying properties make it an excellent herb for cleansing the body. It promotes sweating, which helps the body eliminate toxins (*ama*) and impurities through the skin. Regular use of black pepper supports the liver, kidneys, and digestive system in their detoxification efforts.

Black pepper is also known for its anti-inflammatory effects, which can help reduce joint pain, muscle stiffness, and inflammation associated with conditions such as arthritis. It promotes blood circulation and relieves muscle tension, making it a useful herb for managing chronic pain and inflammation.

Mental Clarity and Cognitive Support

In Ayurveda, black pepper is believed to enhance mental clarity and improve focus. By stimulating the nervous system and increasing circulation, it helps sharpen the mind, improve concentration, and alleviate mental fatigue. Black pepper is sometimes used in herbal formulations to enhance memory and cognitive function.

In summary, black pepper is a vital herb in Ayurvedic medicine, known for its ability to balance the doshas, enhance digestion, stimulate metabolism, support the respiratory and immune systems, and promote detoxification. Its wide range of benefits makes it an essential spice for promoting holistic health and wellness.

Precautions

While black pepper is generally safe in moderate amounts, excessive consumption can cause digestive discomfort and may interact with certain medications. Piperine can increase the absorption of some drugs, so individuals taking medications should consult a healthcare provider before using black pepper in medicinal quantities. Additionally, black pepper should be used sparingly by individuals with acid reflux or stomach ulcers, as its pungency can irritate the digestive tract.

Conclusion

Black pepper is not only a beloved spice in culinary traditions around the world but also a powerful natural remedy with extensive medicinal uses. From enhancing digestion and supporting respiratory health to promoting immunity and improving nutrient absorption, black pepper is a valuable ally for holistic wellness. Its active compound, piperine, amplifies the benefits of other nutrients, making black pepper a unique and essential addition to the diet. By incorporating black pepper into daily meals and herbal remedies, you can harness the numerous health benefits of this humble yet mighty spice, promoting well-being in a natural and flavorful way.

<u>RECIPES</u>

Black pepper (Piper nigrum) is often referred to as the "King of Spices" due to its extensive health benefits, including improving digestion, boosting immunity, and relieving respiratory issues. Here are some medicinal recipes using black pepper:

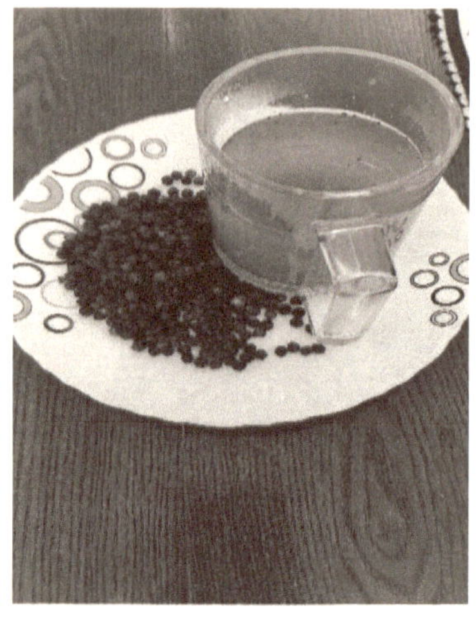

1. Black Pepper Tea for Cold and Cough

Relieves respiratory congestion and soothes sore throat.

Ingredients:

- 1/2 teaspoon black pepper powder

- 1 teaspoon honey

- 1 cup hot water

Instructions:

1. Mix black pepper powder and honey in hot water.

2. Stir well and sip slowly.

3. Drink 2-3 times a day during a cold or cough.

2. Black Pepper and Honey Paste for Cough

Effective for dry or productive cough relief.
Ingredients:

- 1/4 teaspoon black pepper powder

- 1 tablespoon honey

Instructions:

1. Mix black pepper powder with honey to form a paste.

2. Take 1/2 teaspoon 2-3 times daily for cough relief.

3. Black Pepper and Turmeric Milk for Inflammation

Combats inflammation and boosts immunity.
Ingredients:

- 1/4 teaspoon black pepper powder

- 1/2 teaspoon turmeric powder

- 1 cup warm milk

Instructions:

1. Add black pepper and turmeric to warm milk.

2. Stir well and drink before bedtime.

4. Black Pepper Decoction for Digestion

Enhances digestive health and relieves bloating.

Ingredients:

- 1/2 teaspoon black pepper powder

- 1 teaspoon cumin seeds

- 2 cups water

Instructions:

1. Boil water with black pepper and cumin seeds for 5 minutes.

2. Strain and drink warm after meals.

---

5. Black Pepper Oil for Joint Pain Relief

Reduces inflammation and relieves muscle and joint pain.

Ingredients:

- 1/2 teaspoon black pepper powder

- 2 tablespoons coconut oil

Instructions:

1. Heat coconut oil and mix in black pepper powder.

2. Let it cool and massage onto affected areas.

---

6. Black Pepper and Lemon Detox Drink

Boosts metabolism and aids weight loss.

Ingredients:

- 1/4 teaspoon black pepper powder

- Juice of 1/2 lemon

- 1 cup warm water

Instructions:

1. Mix black pepper powder and lemon juice into warm water.

2. Drink in the morning on an empty stomach.

7. Black Pepper Gargle for Sore Throat

Soothes throat irritation and fights infections.
Ingredients:

- 1/2 teaspoon black pepper powder

- 1/2 teaspoon salt

- 1 cup warm water

Instructions:

1. Mix black pepper and salt in warm water.

2. Gargle with this solution 2-3 times a day.

8. Black Pepper and Honey Immunity Booster

Improves immunity and combats fatigue.
Ingredients:

- 1/4 teaspoon black pepper powder

- 1 tablespoon honey

Instructions:

1. Mix black pepper powder with honey.

2. Take 1 teaspoon daily, especially during flu season.

---

9. Black Pepper Steam for Congestion

Clears sinuses and eases nasal congestion.
Ingredients:

- 1 teaspoon black pepper powder

- 4 cups hot water

Instructions:

1. Add black pepper powder to a bowl of hot water.

2. Lean over the bowl, cover your head with a towel, and inhale the steam for 5-10 minutes.

---

10. Black Pepper and Garlic Soup for Immunity

Strengthens immunity and provides warmth during cold weather.
Ingredients:

- 1/2 teaspoon black pepper powder

- 2-3 garlic cloves, chopped

- 1 cup vegetable or chicken broth

Instructions:

1. Boil broth and add garlic and black pepper.

2. Simmer for 10 minutes and drink warm.

These recipes showcase black pepper's versatility and its ability to address various health concerns naturally. Always consult a healthcare provider if you're using black pepper as a remedy alongside medications or for chronic health issues.

Common Myths and Misconceptions About Black Pepper

Black pepper, often referred to as the "king of spices," is one of the most widely used spices in the world, treasured for its pungent flavor and health benefits. However, several myths and misconceptions have emerged around this humble spice. Let's clear up the confusion and explore the truth behind black pepper's many attributes.

---

1. Black Pepper is Just a Culinary Spice

Myth: Black pepper is only useful for enhancing the flavor of food.

Reality: While black pepper is commonly used in cooking, it is also a powerful medicinal herb with a long history in traditional medicine. It has antioxidant, anti-inflammatory, digestive, and even anticancer properties that go beyond just flavoring dishes.

---

2. Black Pepper Has No Health Benefits

Myth: Black pepper is just a simple spice with no real health benefits.

Reality: Black pepper contains piperine, a compound that has been shown to improve digestion, boost metabolism, enhance nutrient absorption, support brain function, and even have anti-inflammatory effects. It's much more than just a flavor enhancer.

3. All Black Pepper is the Same

Myth: There's no difference between varieties of black pepper. **Reality:** While the peppercorns may look similar, the quality of black pepper can vary significantly. The best black pepper comes from regions like Kerala in India. Additionally, the freshness of the pepper and how it's stored can also impact its potency and health benefits.

4. Black Pepper Should Be Consumed in Large Quantities for Maximum Benefit

Myth: The more black pepper you consume, the greater the health benefits. **Reality:** While black pepper has many health benefits, consuming it in excess can irritate the digestive system, leading to issues like acid reflux or stomach upset. A moderate amount—usually 1/4 to 1/2 teaspoon per day—is sufficient to enjoy its benefits.

5. Black Pepper is Dangerous for People with High Blood Pressure

Myth: People with high blood pressure should avoid black pepper. **Reality:** In moderate amounts, black pepper has a beneficial effect on blood pressure. Piperine, the active compound in black pepper, has been shown to help lower blood pressure and improve blood circulation, making it safe for most people with hypertension.

6. Black Pepper Can Replace Prescription Medications

Myth: Black pepper can replace pharmaceutical drugs for various health conditions.

Reality: While black pepper has many health benefits, it should not be used as a substitute for medical treatments or prescription medications. It can be a helpful supplement to a healthy lifestyle but should not be relied upon as a sole treatment for serious health conditions.

7. Black Pepper Can Be Used as a Cure for Cold and Cough

Myth: Black pepper is a guaranteed cure for colds and coughs.
Reality: Black pepper does help alleviate symptoms like congestion and cough by acting as a natural decongestant and expectorant. However, it is not a cure-all for viral infections. It can help ease symptoms, but proper medical treatment is still necessary for full recovery.

8. Black Pepper is Safe for Everyone in Any Form

Myth: Black pepper is safe for everyone and can be consumed in any form.
Reality: While black pepper is safe for most people, some individuals may experience allergic reactions or digestive

discomfort, especially if they consume it in large amounts. People with certain conditions, such as ulcers or gastritis, may need to limit their intake.

9. Black Pepper is Only Effective When Ground

Myth: Only ground black pepper is effective for medicinal use.
Reality: While ground black pepper is commonly used, whole black peppercorns also contain piperine and other compounds that provide health benefits. However, the body absorbs piperine better when black pepper is freshly ground or when it's combined with other foods like turmeric (which increases its absorption).

10. Black Pepper is Bad for Your Stomach

Myth: Black pepper is harsh on the stomach and should be avoided by people with digestive issues.
Reality: While black pepper can irritate the stomach in large quantities, moderate amounts can improve digestion. It stimulates the stomach to produce hydrochloric acid, which aids in breaking down food and improving nutrient absorption. For those with sensitive stomachs, it's important to consume it in moderation.

By dispelling these myths, it's clear that black pepper is not only a flavorful addition to meals but also a powerhouse of health benefits. When used appropriately, it can enhance your well-being and bring a spice of life to both your cooking and your health regimen.

Chapter 9: Cardamom – The Queen of Spices

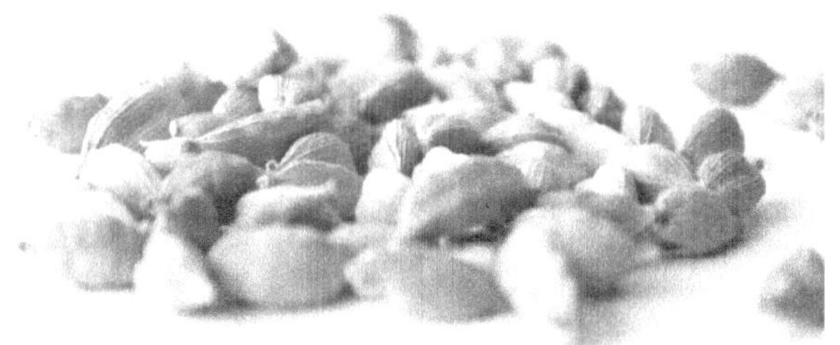

Introduction

Cardamom, often called the "Queen of Spices," is a fragrant spice with a long history of culinary and medicinal use. Known as *Elaichi* in Hindi, cardamom is derived from the seeds of the *Elettaria cardamomum* plant, native to the Indian subcontinent. Its warm, sweet, and slightly citrusy flavor has made it popular in both sweet and savory dishes, but cardamom's true power lies in its medicinal properties. In traditional medicine, especially Ayurveda, cardamom has been used for centuries to treat various ailments, from digestive issues to respiratory problems.

In this chapter, we explore the medicinal importance of cardamom and its role in promoting digestive health, balancing blood sugar, enhancing heart health, and supporting mental well-being. Known for its antioxidant, anti-inflammatory, and antibacterial properties, cardamom offers a range of natural benefits that can improve health and well-being.

Medicinal Importance of Cardamom

Cardamom is rich in essential oils, vitamins, and minerals that contribute to its numerous health benefits. Here's how cardamom can support wellness and address common health issues:

1. Aids Digestive Health

Cardamom is widely regarded as a natural digestive aid, often used to relieve indigestion, bloating, gas, and stomach cramps. Its carminative properties help soothe the digestive tract, improve appetite, and promote the secretion of digestive enzymes, making it effective for overall digestive health.

- **Digestive Tonic**: Adding a pinch of ground cardamom to tea or warm water can alleviate bloating, reduce acidity, and relieve stomach discomfort after meals.

HEALTH BENEFITS OF CARDAMOM

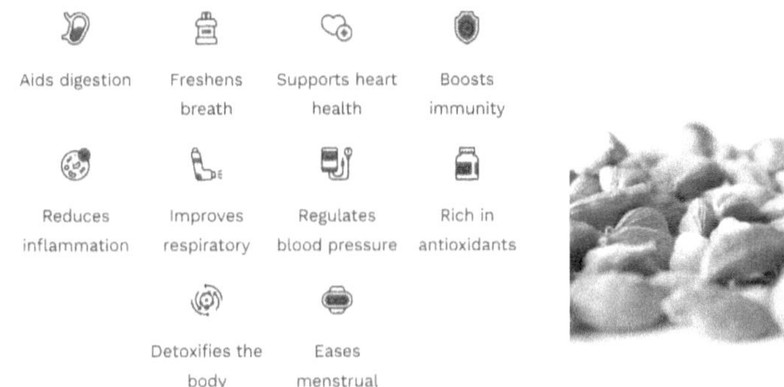

2. Balances Blood Sugar Levels

Studies suggest that cardamom may help regulate blood sugar levels, making it beneficial for individuals with diabetes or those looking to manage blood sugar naturally. Compounds in cardamom help improve insulin sensitivity, which can aid in controlling blood sugar spikes.

- **Blood Sugar Support**: Incorporating cardamom into meals or beverages can help keep blood sugar levels stable, especially when consumed with other blood sugar-supporting foods.

3. Supports Heart Health

Cardamom has been shown to have a positive impact on heart health. Its antioxidant properties help protect against oxidative stress, which can contribute to heart disease. Additionally, cardamom may help lower blood pressure by acting as a natural diuretic and reducing stress, which also supports heart health.

- **Heart Health**: Drinking cardamom-infused tea can be a gentle way to support healthy blood pressure and reduce the risk of heart-related issues over time.

4. Powerful Antioxidant

Cardamom is rich in antioxidants, which help neutralize harmful free radicals and reduce oxidative stress in the body. These antioxidants play a role in protecting cells from damage and reducing the risk of chronic diseases, including certain cancers.

- **Daily Antioxidant Boost**: Including cardamom in smoothies, teas, or meals can enhance antioxidant intake, supporting cellular health and reducing the effects of aging.

5. Enhances Respiratory Health

Cardamom's essential oils have a warming effect, which can help alleviate respiratory issues such as cough, cold, and asthma. Cardamom acts as an expectorant, helping to loosen mucus and clear airways, making it easier to breathe. Its antibacterial properties also help fight respiratory infections.

- **Respiratory Relief**: Drinking warm cardamom tea can soothe a sore throat, relieve cough, and help open up congested airways, making it beneficial for colds and bronchitis.

6. Improves Oral Health

Due to its antibacterial properties, cardamom is often used as a natural remedy for oral health. It helps fight bacteria that cause bad breath and protects against infections in the mouth.

In many cultures, chewing on cardamom pods is a traditional practice to freshen breath.

- **Natural Breath Freshener**: Chewing on a cardamom pod after meals can help maintain oral hygiene, freshen breath, and protect the mouth from bacterial buildup.

7. Promotes Mental Clarity and Reduces Anxiety

In traditional medicine, cardamom is valued for its ability to enhance mental clarity, relieve anxiety, and promote relaxation. The essential oils in cardamom can act as mild antidepressants, helping to reduce stress and improve mood. Aromatherapy with cardamom oil is known to help alleviate anxiety and promote a sense of calm.

- **Stress Relief**: Sipping cardamom tea or using cardamom essential oil in a diffuser can provide a soothing effect on the mind, helping to reduce anxiety and enhance mental clarity.

8. Anti-Inflammatory Properties

Cardamom contains compounds with anti-inflammatory effects, which can help reduce inflammation throughout the body. This is particularly beneficial for individuals with chronic inflammatory conditions like arthritis. By reducing inflammatory markers, cardamom can help alleviate joint pain and promote mobility.

- **Joint Health**: Adding cardamom to meals or herbal teas may help manage inflammation and reduce pain for those with arthritis or similar inflammatory conditions.

9. Supports Detoxification

Cardamom acts as a natural diuretic, helping the body flush out toxins through increased urine output. This detoxifying effect supports kidney health and aids in the removal of waste products from the body, promoting a cleaner internal system.

- **Detox Drink**: Adding cardamom to herbal teas or warm lemon water can support the kidneys in flushing out toxins, promoting overall detoxification.

10. Boosts Immunity

Cardamom is a natural immune booster thanks to its antibacterial, antiviral, and antioxidant properties. These qualities make cardamom effective in fighting infections and strengthening the body's defenses, particularly during times when the immune system is vulnerable, like flu season.

- **Immunity Tea**: Cardamom tea with honey and ginger is a comforting way to boost immunity, soothe the throat, and prevent respiratory infections.

Incorporating Cardamom into Daily Life

Cardamom can be used in a variety of ways to promote health:

- **Cardamom Tea**: Boil cardamom pods with water, add honey or ginger for added benefits, and enjoy this fragrant tea for digestive and respiratory health.

- **Cooking**: Add cardamom to curries, stews, desserts, and rice dishes to enhance flavor and boost health benefits.

- **Chewing**: Chewing on cardamom pods can freshen breath, improve digestion, and calm the mind.

Ayurvedic Context of Cardamom

Cardamom (*Elettaria cardamomum*), known as *Ela* in Sanskrit, is one of Ayurveda's most cherished and versatile spices. Often referred to as the "queen of spices," cardamom has a rich history of use in Ayurvedic medicine for its cooling, soothing, and revitalizing properties. With its sweet, aromatic flavor, it is used not only as a culinary spice but also as a medicinal herb, offering a wide range of therapeutic benefits for the mind and body.

Dosha Balancing Properties

Cardamom is considered a *Tridoshic* herb, meaning it has the unique ability to balance all three doshas—*Vata*, *Pitta*, and *Kapha*. It has a cooling (*sheeta*) energy and a sweet (*madhura*) taste, making it especially effective in calming the heat associated with *Pitta* imbalances. Its light (*laghu*) and aromatic qualities help balance *Vata* and *Kapha*, particularly when there are issues like congestion, bloating, or digestive sluggishness.

Cardamom is often recommended for individuals who experience digestive discomfort due to excessive heat or acidity (typically a *Pitta* imbalance), as well as for those dealing with *Vata*-related digestive irregularities like bloating and gas.

Digestive and Detoxification Support

One of cardamom's most important uses in Ayurveda is for its digestive properties. It stimulates the digestive fire (*Agni*), improving the metabolism and enhancing the body's ability to digest food. Cardamom is commonly used to relieve indigestion, gas, bloating, and nausea. It also helps to soothe an upset stomach and is often included in Ayurvedic formulations for digestive health.

Cardamom's detoxifying properties support the body's natural cleansing processes, especially in eliminating toxins (*ama*) that may accumulate due to poor digestion. It helps purify the blood and maintain the health of the digestive organs, including the liver and intestines.

Respiratory and Immune Support

Cardamom is highly effective in promoting respiratory health. Its aromatic and expectorant properties help to clear mucus, open the airways, and relieve congestion. It is often used in Ayurvedic remedies for coughs, asthma, bronchitis, and other respiratory issues. A traditional treatment involves chewing on cardamom pods or adding it to warm tea to soothe the throat and improve breathing.

The spice is also a potent immune booster. Its antioxidant-rich compounds help fight free radicals, supporting the immune system and promoting overall vitality. By boosting circulation and promoting good digestion, cardamom strengthens the body's ability to resist illness.

Mental Clarity and Stress Relief

Cardamom is considered a natural mood enhancer in Ayurveda. Its uplifting properties support mental clarity and focus, making it beneficial for cognitive health. It is also used to relieve stress, anxiety, and emotional tension. The sweet, warm aroma of cardamom has a calming effect on the mind, reducing mental fatigue and promoting a sense of peace and well-being.

Heart and Circulatory Health

Cardamom is also known for its cardiovascular benefits. It helps to improve circulation, reduce high blood pressure, and promote heart health by supporting the smooth flow of blood. It is a mild diuretic, helping to eliminate excess fluid and toxins from the body, which can reduce the burden on the heart and kidneys.

In summary, cardamom is a highly valued herb in Ayurveda for its wide-ranging benefits. It enhances digestion, detoxifies the body, promotes respiratory and immune health, and supports mental clarity. Its ability to balance all three doshas makes it an indispensable component in maintaining overall health and harmony. Whether used in cooking, teas, or as part of Ayurvedic formulations, cardamom offers both physical and emotional nourishment.

Precautions

Cardamom is generally safe in moderate amounts, but overconsumption may cause mild side effects, such as digestive discomfort in sensitive individuals. People with gallstones should avoid high quantities of cardamom, as it can stimulate bile production. Pregnant and breastfeeding women should consult a healthcare provider before using cardamom medicinally.

Conclusion

Cardamom is not only a beloved spice in global cuisines but also a powerful remedy with extensive medicinal benefits. Its unique combination of digestive, antioxidant, anti-inflammatory, and antibacterial properties makes it a valuable addition to a holistic wellness routine. By incorporating cardamom into daily meals, teas, or natural remedies, you can enjoy the numerous health benefits it has to offer. From supporting digestion and respiratory health to promoting mental clarity and detoxification, cardamom truly lives up to its title as the "Queen of Spices."

<u>RECIPES</u>

Cardamom (Elettaria cardamomum), often referred to as the "Queen of Spices," is renowned for its digestive, respiratory, and anti-inflammatory properties. Below are some effective medicinal recipes using cardamom:

---

1. Cardamom Tea for Digestion

Improves digestion and relieves bloating.
Ingredients:

- 2-3 cardamom pods (crushed)

- 1 teaspoon grated ginger (optional)

- 1 cup water

Instructions:

1. Boil water and add crushed cardamom pods and ginger.

2. Simmer for 5-7 minutes.

3. Strain and drink warm after meals.

---

2. Cardamom Milk for Better Sleep

Promotes relaxation and improves sleep quality.
Ingredients:

- 1/4 teaspoon cardamom powder

- 1 cup warm milk

- Honey (optional)

Instructions:

1. Mix cardamom powder into warm milk.

2. Add honey if desired, and drink before bedtime.

---

3. Cardamom and Honey Cough Remedy

Relieves cough and soothes the throat.
Ingredients:

- 1/4 teaspoon cardamom powder

- 1 tablespoon honey

Instructions:

1. Mix cardamom powder with honey.

2. Take 1 teaspoon twice daily for relief.

---

4. Cardamom Detox Water

Flushes toxins and supports kidney health.
Ingredients:

- 2-3 cardamom pods

- 1 liter water

Instructions:

1. Slightly crush the cardamom pods and add them to water.

2. Let it infuse overnight.

3. Drink throughout the day.

5. Cardamom and Cinnamon Tea for Respiratory Health

Eases congestion and supports lung function.
Ingredients:

- 2-3 cardamom pods (crushed)

- 1 stick of cinnamon

- 1 cup water

Instructions:

1. Boil water with cardamom and cinnamon.

2. Simmer for 10 minutes and strain.

3. Drink warm for respiratory relief.

6. Cardamom Face Mask for Glowing Skin

Improves skin texture and reduces blemishes.
Ingredients:

- 1/4 teaspoon cardamom powder

- 1 tablespoon honey

- 1 teaspoon yogurt

Instructions:

1. Mix cardamom powder with honey and yogurt.

2. Apply to the face and leave on for 15 minutes.

3. Rinse with warm water.

---

7. Cardamom Water for Bad Breath

Freshens breath and fights oral bacteria.
Ingredients:

- 2 cardamom pods

- 1 cup warm water

Instructions:

1. Crush cardamom pods and add to warm water.

2. Use as a mouth rinse after meals.

---

8. Cardamom Infused Coffee for Energy Boost

Enhances mood and provides an energy boost.
Ingredients:

- 1/4 teaspoon cardamom powder

- 1 cup brewed coffee

Instructions:

1. Add cardamom powder to freshly brewed coffee.

2. Stir well and enjoy.

---

9. Cardamom and Turmeric Golden Milk

Reduces inflammation and boosts immunity.
Ingredients:

- 1/4 teaspoon cardamom powder

- 1/2 teaspoon turmeric powder

- 1 cup warm milk

Instructions:

1. Mix cardamom and turmeric into warm milk.

2. Drink daily for overall health benefits.

---

10. Cardamom Oil for Muscle Pain Relief

Eases muscle tension and improves circulation.
Ingredients:

- 5-6 drops cardamom essential oil

- 2 tablespoons carrier oil (coconut or olive oil)

Instructions:

1. Mix cardamom essential oil with the carrier oil.

2. Massage onto sore muscles as needed.

These recipes showcase cardamom's versatility and its natural ability to address various health concerns. As with all remedies, consult a healthcare provider for specific health conditions or if you are on medications.

Common Myths and Misconceptions About Cardamom

Cardamom, often referred to as the "queen of spices," is one of the most prized and aromatic spices in the world. Known for its distinctive flavor and many health benefits, cardamom has become a staple in both cooking and traditional medicine. However, several myths and misconceptions have emerged around this flavorful spice. Let's separate fact from fiction about cardamom.

1. All Cardamom Is the Same

Myth: All varieties of cardamom are the same in taste and medicinal value.

Reality: There are two main types of cardamom: **green cardamom** and **black cardamom**. Green cardamom is sweeter, floral, and more aromatic, while black cardamom has a smoky, earthy flavor. They have different uses in cooking and medicine, with green cardamom being more common in sweet dishes and teas, while black cardamom is used in savory dishes. Both have distinct health benefits.

2. Cardamom Can Cure All Stomach Issues

Myth: Cardamom is a miracle cure for all digestive problems.

Reality: While cardamom can certainly help improve digestion and relieve bloating or indigestion, it is not a cure for all gastrointestinal conditions. It can aid in soothing mild stomach issues like gas and nausea but may not resolve more serious conditions like ulcers, chronic acidity, or IBS. It's best used as part of an overall digestive health plan.

3. Cardamom Is Only Used in Sweets and Desserts

Myth: Cardamom is only a flavoring agent for sweet foods and desserts.

Reality: While cardamom is often found in desserts and drinks like chai or rice pudding, it is also widely used in savory dishes, especially in Middle Eastern, Indian, and Scandinavian cuisines. It enhances the flavor of curries, stews, and meats and can be used in spice blends like garam masala. Its versatility in both sweet and savory dishes makes it an essential spice.

4. Cardamom Is Expensive and Not Worth the Price

Myth: Cardamom is too expensive for the benefits it offers.

Reality: While cardamom is one of the more expensive spices, it offers a wealth of benefits that make it worth the price. Its medicinal properties, including its ability to soothe digestive issues, reduce inflammation, improve oral health, and even reduce anxiety, make it a valuable addition to any kitchen or wellness routine. Its potent flavor also means you need very little to enhance a dish.

5. Cardamom Is Safe for Everyone

Myth: Cardamom is harmless and can be consumed by anyone.

Reality: While cardamom is generally safe for most people, excessive consumption can cause allergic reactions or digestive discomfort in some individuals. People with known allergies to spices or individuals who are pregnant should consult their healthcare provider before using cardamom in large quantities or as a supplement.

6. Cardamom Is Only Effective When Used Fresh

Myth: Cardamom loses all its medicinal benefits once it is dried or ground.

Reality: While freshly ground cardamom does have the most intense flavor and aroma, dried and ground cardamom still retains its health benefits. The key is to store it in an airtight container, away from light and moisture, to maintain its potency. Whether whole or ground, cardamom continues to provide digestive, anti-inflammatory, and antioxidant benefits.

7. Cardamom Can Instantly Relieve Bad Breath

Myth: Cardamom is an instant cure for bad breath and can eliminate it permanently.

Reality: Cardamom can temporarily freshen breath due to its antibacterial properties, but it's not a permanent solution for bad breath (halitosis). The underlying cause of bad breath, such as poor oral hygiene, gum disease, or digestive issues, should be addressed for long-term relief. Cardamom can be part of an oral health regimen but is not a replacement for proper dental care.

8. Cardamom Can Be Used to Replace All Other Spices

Myth: Cardamom can replace any other spice in a recipe.
Reality: While cardamom has a unique flavor profile, it does not work as a replacement for all spices. Its distinct taste may overpower other ingredients if used excessively. It pairs well with spices like cinnamon, cloves, and nutmeg, but should not be used as a substitute for spices that bring different flavor notes (like cumin, turmeric, or chili).

9. Cardamom Should Only Be Consumed as a Tea

Myth: The best way to consume cardamom is in tea.
Reality: While cardamom tea is an excellent way to enjoy its health benefits, cardamom can be consumed in many forms, including as a spice in cooking, added to smoothies, or as part of herbal remedies. You can also chew on cardamom seeds for a quick digestive aid or use them in oil infusions.

10. Cardamom is Harmful to People with High Blood Pressure

Myth: Cardamom increases blood pressure and should be avoided by those with hypertension.
Reality: In fact, cardamom has been shown to help reduce

blood pressure. It contains compounds that improve circulation and help relax blood vessels. Regular consumption of cardamom, in moderate amounts, may actually benefit people with high blood pressure as part of a balanced, heart-healthy diet.

By debunking these myths, we can better appreciate cardamom's true value—not only as a flavorful spice but as a powerhouse of health benefits. Whether used in cooking, beverages, or for medicinal purposes, cardamom continues to hold a special place in both traditional and modern wellness practices.

Chapter 10: Fennel – The Soothing Digestive

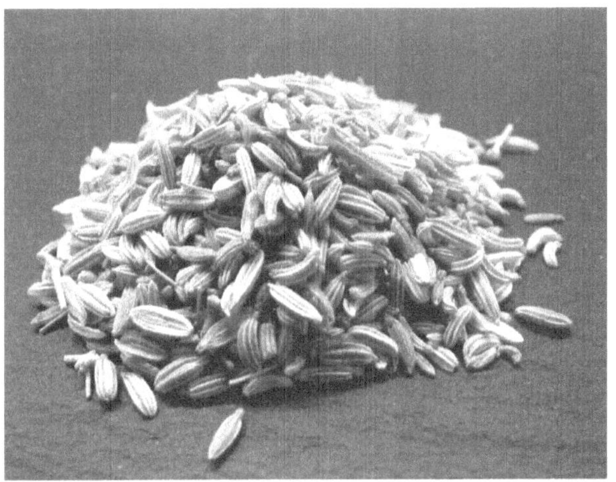

Introduction

Fennel, known as *Saunf* in Hindi, is a versatile spice recognized for its sweet, licorice-like flavor and distinct aroma. This seed, derived from the *Foeniculum vulgare* plant, is widely used in Indian cuisine, often enjoyed after meals as a natural mouth freshener and digestive aid. Beyond its culinary uses, fennel has a long history in traditional medicine, valued for its ability to soothe digestion, improve respiratory health, and balance hormones. Packed with essential nutrients, antioxidants, and bioactive compounds, fennel is celebrated for its natural healing abilities.

In this chapter, we delve into the medicinal benefits of fennel and how its gentle yet effective properties make it a staple for promoting health. Known for aiding digestion, supporting hormonal balance, and acting as a natural detoxifier, fennel seeds offer a wide range of therapeutic benefits that make them a valuable addition to the Indian kitchen and natural medicine cabinet.

Medicinal Importance of Fennel

Fennel is rich in fiber, vitamins, and antioxidants, which contribute to its therapeutic effects. Here are some of the ways fennel can support health and help with various ailments:

1. Improves Digestive Health

One of fennel's most well-known benefits is its ability to support digestive health. Fennel seeds contain compounds that relax the gastrointestinal muscles, helping alleviate bloating, gas, and indigestion. Its carminative and anti-spasmodic properties make it effective in soothing the digestive tract and reducing discomfort.

- **Digestive Tonic**: Chewing on fennel seeds after meals or brewing them into a tea can help relieve indigestion, reduce bloating, and promote a smoother digestive process.

HEALTH BENEFITS OF FENNEL

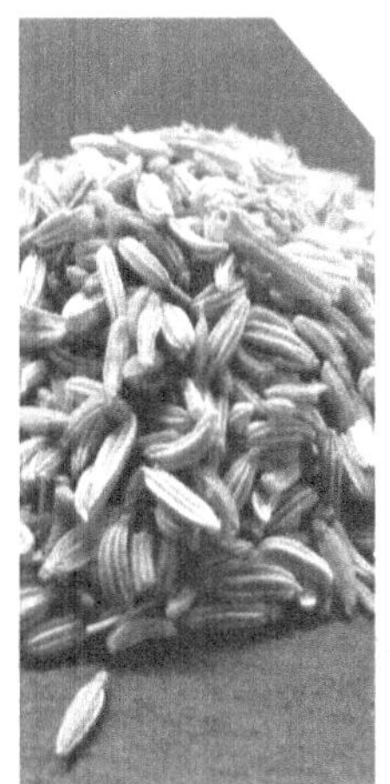

Aids digestion

Relieves bloating

Supports heart health

Improves eyesight

Boosts immunity

Regulates blood pressure

Eases menstrual pain

Rich in antioxidants

Promotes liver health

Freshens breath

2. Natural Remedy for Acid Reflux

Fennel's alkaline nature helps in reducing acidity in the stomach, making it a helpful remedy for acid reflux. Fennel also supports the secretion of digestive enzymes, reducing the risk of heartburn and other symptoms associated with high acidity.

- **Acid Relief**: A warm fennel tea or a few seeds after meals can help balance stomach acid, soothe the stomach lining, and provide relief from acid reflux.

3. Anti-Inflammatory Properties

Fennel contains antioxidants like flavonoids and phenolic compounds, which help reduce inflammation in the body. Chronic inflammation is linked to many diseases, including arthritis, heart disease, and diabetes, and fennel's natural anti-inflammatory properties make it beneficial for overall health.

- **Joint Health**: Consuming fennel regularly can help reduce inflammation and alleviate symptoms in individuals suffering from inflammatory conditions, such as arthritis.

4. Promotes Hormonal Balance

In traditional medicine, fennel has been used as a natural remedy to help balance hormones. It contains phytoestrogens, which are plant compounds that mimic estrogen in the body, making it particularly beneficial for women's health. Fennel can help regulate menstrual cycles, reduce menopausal symptoms, and support hormonal balance.

- **Women's Health**: Drinking fennel tea may help relieve menstrual discomfort, balance hormones, and support reproductive health in women.

5. Supports Respiratory Health

Fennel has mild expectorant properties, which make it useful for clearing respiratory congestion and easing breathing. Its anti-inflammatory and antibacterial properties also help fight respiratory infections and support overall lung health.

- **Respiratory Aid**: A warm fennel tea can help soothe a sore throat, reduce cough, and provide relief from cold symptoms by loosening mucus and supporting clearer airways.

6. Natural Detoxifier

Fennel is a natural diuretic, meaning it helps increase urine output and supports the body's detoxification processes. By promoting the removal of toxins through urine, fennel aids kidney function and helps keep the body clean from unwanted waste products.

- **Detox Drink**: Consuming fennel tea regularly can help flush out toxins, supporting kidney health and aiding in the body's natural detoxification.

7. Rich in Antioxidants

Fennel seeds are packed with antioxidants that protect cells from oxidative stress and free radical damage. These antioxidants, including vitamin C and flavonoids, play a role in reducing the risk of chronic diseases and slowing the effects of aging.

- **Antioxidant Boost**: Adding fennel to daily meals or drinking fennel tea can enhance antioxidant intake and support the body's defenses against cell damage.

8. Improves Vision and Eye Health

Fennel contains vitamin A and other antioxidants that support eye health. It has been used in traditional remedies to improve vision and alleviate eye strain, especially due to its high nutrient content and anti-inflammatory properties.

- **Eye Health Tip**: Drinking fennel tea or using it in dishes can provide beneficial nutrients that support eye health and protect against vision-related issues.

9. Supports Weight Management

The high fiber content in fennel seeds promotes a feeling of fullness, which can help control appetite and prevent overeating. Fennel also stimulates metabolism and can aid in reducing water retention, making it beneficial for those aiming to manage or reduce body weight.

- **Weight Management**: Drinking fennel water in the morning can aid in weight loss by reducing cravings and promoting fat metabolism.

10. Boosts Immune System

Fennel's antioxidant and antibacterial properties make it a natural immune booster. It supports the body in fighting off infections, particularly in the respiratory and digestive tracts. The high vitamin C content in fennel also helps strengthen immune defenses, keeping the body resilient against illnesses.

- **Immunity Tea**: Regularly consuming fennel tea with honey can help boost immunity, especially during cold and flu season, supporting the body's natural defenses.

Incorporating Fennel into Daily Life

Fennel can be used in a variety of ways to promote health:

- **Fennel Tea**: Boil fennel seeds in water to make a soothing tea, helpful for digestion, detoxification, and immune support.

- **Cooking**: Add fennel seeds to curries, soups, or rice dishes to enhance flavor and gain health benefits.

- **Mouth Freshener**: Chewing fennel seeds after meals is a traditional way to freshen breath and support digestion.

225

Ayurvedic Context of Fennel

Fennel (*Foeniculum vulgare*), known as *Saunf* in Sanskrit, is a highly regarded herb in Ayurveda for its cooling, soothing, and digestive-enhancing properties. It is celebrated for its sweet, aromatic flavor and numerous therapeutic benefits, making it a staple in both Ayurvedic medicine and Indian cuisine. In Ayurveda, fennel is considered a powerful tool for balancing the doshas, especially *Vata* and *Pitta*, and is used to promote digestive health, support detoxification, and soothe various ailments.

Dosha Balancing Properties

Fennel is primarily known for its ability to balance *Vata* and *Pitta* doshas due to its sweet (*madhura*) and slightly pungent (*katu*) taste, as well as its cooling (*sheeta*) energy. Its warming and stimulating properties help regulate *Vata*, making it beneficial for alleviating bloating, gas, and digestive irregularities. Fennel also helps soothe excess heat and inflammation caused by *Pitta* imbalances, making it ideal for individuals prone to acidity, indigestion, and digestive discomfort.

Fennel is considered very gentle and is typically safe for all constitutions, though it is especially recommended for those with *Vata* and *Pitta* imbalances. It can be used regularly to maintain balance and harmony in the body.

Digestive Support

In Ayurveda, fennel is highly valued for its potent digestive benefits. It is known to stimulate *Agni* (digestive fire), helping to promote the proper breakdown of food and nutrients.

Fennel seeds are often chewed after meals to improve digestion, alleviate bloating, and relieve indigestion. It is also effective in reducing excessive gas and flatulence, making it an ideal remedy for digestive discomfort.

Fennel is a carminative, meaning it helps prevent the formation of gas in the digestive tract and encourages the smooth movement of food through the intestines. It is frequently used in Ayurvedic herbal blends to enhance digestion and promote a healthy, efficient digestive system.

Detoxification and Liver Health

Fennel supports the body's natural detoxification process by aiding in the elimination of toxins (*ama*) through its diuretic and antioxidant properties. It promotes the health of the liver and kidneys, supporting their detoxifying functions. Fennel is commonly used in Ayurvedic treatments to cleanse the body and purify the blood, helping to maintain overall health and vitality.

Respiratory Health

Fennel is also beneficial for the respiratory system, particularly in alleviating congestion, coughing, and sinusitis. Its mild expectorant properties help loosen mucus in the lungs and ease breathing. Fennel is often used in Ayurvedic formulations to treat respiratory issues such as asthma, bronchitis, and cold-related coughs.

Hormonal Balance and Women's Health

Fennel is especially revered for its ability to support hormonal balance, particularly in women. It is considered an effective herb for relieving menstrual discomfort, regulating the menstrual cycle, and alleviating symptoms associated with menopause. Fennel seeds contain phytoestrogens, which help to balance estrogen levels in the body, promoting overall reproductive health.

In addition, fennel is used to promote lactation in nursing mothers by increasing milk production. A warm fennel tea is often recommended to support breastfeeding mothers and enhance milk supply.

Mental Clarity and Stress Relief

Fennel is also valued for its calming and uplifting properties, which make it beneficial for mental clarity and emotional well-being. It is often used to alleviate stress, anxiety, and nervous tension, providing a sense of peace and relaxation. Fennel is known to support clear thinking and enhance cognitive function, making it a valuable herb for maintaining mental sharpness.

In summary, fennel is a versatile and highly effective herb in Ayurveda, offering a wide array of health benefits. It supports digestive health, detoxifies the body, promotes respiratory well-being, balances hormones, and soothes the mind. Whether used as a spice, tea, or in Ayurvedic formulations, fennel plays an essential role in maintaining balance, harmony, and vitality in the body.

Precautions

While fennel is generally safe for most people, excessive consumption should be avoided, as it may lead to mild side effects such as nausea. Pregnant women should consult a healthcare provider before using fennel medicinally due to its phytoestrogen content, which may interfere with hormonal balance. Individuals with allergies to celery, carrots, or other plants in the Apiaceae family should also exercise caution.

Conclusion

Fennel is a staple in the Indian kitchen and a versatile medicinal spice that offers numerous health benefits. From aiding digestion and balancing hormones to supporting respiratory health and boosting immunity, fennel's therapeutic properties make it an essential addition to daily life. Its gentle and effective action makes it a valuable remedy for a range of ailments, offering natural support for both physical and mental well-being. By incorporating fennel into daily meals, teas, and natural remedies, you can take advantage of its powerful health benefits and experience the comfort and relief it brings.

<u>RECIPES</u>

Fennel (Foeniculum vulgare) is a fragrant herb known for its digestive, anti-inflammatory, and antioxidant properties. It is commonly used to address gastrointestinal issues, boost immunity, and support overall health. Below are some medicinal recipes using fennel:

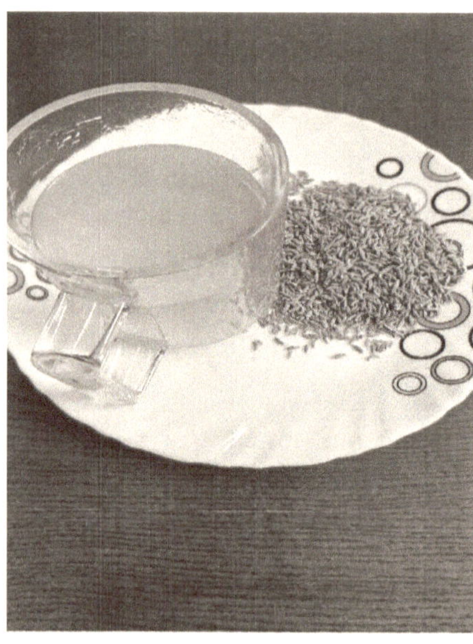

1. Fennel Tea for Digestion

Relieves bloating, gas, and indigestion.

Ingredients:

- 1 teaspoon fennel seeds

- 1 cup boiling water

Instructions:

1. Crush fennel seeds lightly to release oils.

2. Steep in boiling water for 10 minutes.

3. Strain and drink warm after meals.

---

2. Fennel Water for Detox

Supports detoxification and kidney health.
Ingredients:

- 1 tablespoon fennel seeds

- 1 liter water

Instructions:

1. Boil water and add fennel seeds.

2. Let it cool and strain.

3. Drink throughout the day.

3. Fennel and Honey Cough Remedy

Eases cough and soothes sore throat.
Ingredients:

- 1 teaspoon fennel seed powder

- 1 tablespoon honey

Instructions:

1. Mix fennel powder with honey.

2. Take 1 teaspoon twice daily to alleviate cough.

4. Fennel Infusion for Menstrual Cramps

Reduces pain and discomfort during menstruation.
Ingredients:

- 1 teaspoon fennel seeds

- 1 cup hot water

Instructions:

1. Steep fennel seeds in hot water for 10 minutes.

2. Strain and drink warm during cramps.

5. Fennel Seed Gargle for Bad Breath

Freshens breath and fights oral bacteria.
Ingredients:

- 1 teaspoon fennel seeds

- 1 cup warm water

Instructions:

1. Boil fennel seeds in water for 5 minutes.

2. Strain and let it cool slightly.

3. Use as a gargle after meals.

6. Fennel and Ginger Tea for Nausea

Relieves nausea and improves digestion.
Ingredients:

- 1 teaspoon fennel seeds

- 1/2 teaspoon grated ginger

- 1 cup boiling water

Instructions:

1. Combine fennel seeds and ginger in boiling water.

2. Steep for 10 minutes, strain, and drink warm.

7. Fennel Seed Powder for Constipation

Acts as a mild laxative and improves bowel movement.
Ingredients:

- 1 teaspoon fennel seed powder

- 1 glass warm water

Instructions:

1. Mix fennel seed powder into warm water.

2. Drink on an empty stomach in the morning.

8. Fennel and Cardamom Tea for Bloating

Reduces gas and soothes stomach discomfort.
Ingredients:

- 1 teaspoon fennel seeds

- 2 crushed cardamom pods

- 1 cup boiling water

Instructions:

1. Add fennel seeds and cardamom to boiling water.

2. Steep for 10 minutes, strain, and enjoy.

9. Fennel and Honey Syrup for Immunity

Boosts immunity and reduces inflammation.
Ingredients:

- 2 teaspoons fennel seeds
- 1 tablespoon honey
- 1 cup water

Instructions:

1. Boil fennel seeds in water until reduced to half.
2. Strain and mix with honey.
3. Take 1 tablespoon daily.

---

10. Fennel Poultice for Eye Strain

Soothes tired or irritated eyes.
Ingredients:

- 1 teaspoon fennel seeds
- 1 cup water

Instructions:

1. Boil fennel seeds in water and let it cool.
2. Soak a clean cloth in the liquid and place it over closed eyes for 10 minutes.

These fennel-based recipes highlight its versatility and natural healing properties. Always consult a healthcare provider before using fennel remedies if you have underlying health conditions or are on medication.

Common Myths and Misconceptions About Fennel

Fennel, a fragrant and flavorful herb, has long been celebrated for its culinary and medicinal uses. From fresh fennel bulbs to fennel seeds, this versatile plant has many health benefits. However, there are also several myths and misconceptions surrounding fennel that can lead to misunderstandings about its use. Let's debunk these common myths and set the record straight!

1. Fennel Is Only Used for Flavoring Dishes

Myth: Fennel is just a flavoring herb with no medicinal properties.

Reality: While fennel is a popular ingredient in cooking, especially in Mediterranean and Indian cuisines, it has significant medicinal value. Fennel seeds are known for their digestive benefits, including reducing bloating, easing indigestion, and acting as a natural diuretic. It also has anti-inflammatory and antioxidant properties.

2. Fennel Is Just for Women

Myth: Fennel is a herb meant specifically for women, especially for menstrual or hormonal issues.

Reality: While fennel does have benefits for women, particularly in regulating menstrual cycles and promoting lactation, it is equally beneficial for men. Fennel can help with digestion, support respiratory health, and even aid in reducing inflammation. It is a versatile herb suitable for all genders.

3. Fennel Is a Strong Laxative

Myth: Fennel is a potent laxative that should be avoided.

Reality: Fennel does have mild laxative properties, but it is not as harsh as other medicinal herbs used for constipation. It helps improve digestion and prevent bloating and gas, which in turn can promote regular bowel movements. In moderation, fennel is safe and effective for promoting digestive health.

4. Fennel Seeds Are Only Used for Digestive Problems

Myth: Fennel seeds are only useful for digestion and nothing else.

Reality: Fennel seeds are not just a digestive aid. They are also packed with antioxidants, vitamin C, fiber, and essential minerals like potassium, calcium, and magnesium. They support heart health, reduce inflammation, improve vision, and have antimicrobial properties. Fennel also supports weight loss by increasing metabolism and controlling appetite.

5. Fennel Can Be Consumed in Unlimited Quantities Without Any Side Effects

Myth: There are no side effects to eating as much fennel as you want.

Reality: While fennel is generally safe for most people, consuming it in excessive amounts can lead to digestive issues like heartburn or gas. People who are allergic to plants in the carrot family (Apiaceae) may also be allergic to fennel. Pregnant women should avoid large quantities of fennel due to its mild estrogenic effects.

6. Fennel Is Only Beneficial When Consumed in Tea

Myth: The only way to get fennel's benefits is by drinking fennel tea.

Reality: Fennel can be consumed in various ways—whether raw (as a crunchy addition to salads), roasted, or in ground form as a spice. Fennel seeds can also be added to curries, soups, stews, and baked goods. The medicinal benefits are present whether you consume fennel as a whole seed, ground powder, or in teas.

7. Fennel Is the Same as Aniseed

Myth: Fennel and aniseed are the same spice.

Reality: Fennel and aniseed are often confused because they share a similar licorice-like flavor. However, they are different plants. Fennel has a milder, sweeter taste and is a member of the Apiaceae family, while aniseed is a member of the Apiaceae but has a stronger, more distinct flavor and is used in different contexts. They are not interchangeable, and fennel is typically more versatile in cooking.

8. Fennel Causes Breast Enlargement in Women

Myth: Fennel causes breast enlargement due to its estrogen-like properties.

Reality: While fennel does contain phytoestrogens (plant-based compounds that mimic estrogen), there is no conclusive evidence to suggest that it causes breast enlargement. Fennel may help with hormonal balance and lactation but should not be relied upon as a breast-enhancing herb. It may help regulate the menstrual cycle and promote milk production in nursing mothers.

9. Fennel Can Cure All Respiratory Issues

Myth: Fennel is a miracle cure for all respiratory issues.

Reality: Fennel does have mild expectorant properties, meaning it can help loosen mucus and ease coughing, which can be useful for treating colds or respiratory congestion. However, it is not a cure-all for serious respiratory conditions like asthma, bronchitis, or pneumonia. It should be used as a complementary remedy, not a replacement for medical treatment.

10. Fennel Is Only Available in Indian or Mediterranean Cuisines

Myth: Fennel is a spice exclusive to Indian or Mediterranean cooking.

Reality: While fennel is certainly a key ingredient in both Indian and Mediterranean cuisine, it is widely used in other parts of the world too. In Western cuisines, fennel is used in Italian sausages, seafood dishes, and as a fresh salad vegetable. Its seeds are also found in many European and Middle Eastern spice blends, such as Italian sausage mix and Chinese five-spice powder.

By debunking these myths, we can fully appreciate the many benefits of fennel, not just as a flavorful spice, but as a valuable medicinal herb. From aiding digestion to supporting overall health, fennel has earned its place in the kitchen and the medicine cabinet, and it's a herb worth including in your daily routine!

Conclusion

The use of medicinal spices in Indian kitchens is a practice deeply rooted in tradition, offering both culinary delight and numerous health benefits. These spices are not just flavor enhancers but powerful natural remedies that support overall well-being. Turmeric's anti-inflammatory and antioxidant properties help combat chronic diseases, while cumin aids digestion and improves gut health. Ginger is widely recognized for its ability to soothe nausea and boost immunity, while cinnamon helps regulate blood sugar and supports heart health. Each of these spices carries unique medicinal properties that contribute to a balanced and holistic lifestyle.

In today's fast-paced world, where processed foods and artificial additives have become the norm, returning to natural, time-tested ingredients is essential. Spices like fenugreek, cloves, cardamom, and mustard seeds provide antimicrobial, anti-inflammatory, and digestive benefits, making them invaluable in promoting long-term health. Modern scientific research continues to validate what ancient Indian medicine has known for centuries—these spices serve as nature's pharmacy, offering protection against various ailments.

Incorporating these spices into daily cooking is a simple and effective way to harness their healing potential. Whether used in curries, teas, or herbal concoctions, they provide a natural defense against illness while enhancing the taste of food. By embracing the wisdom of traditional Indian cooking, we not only nourish our bodies but also preserve a heritage of holistic health. Truly, these kitchen staples demonstrate that food is not just sustenance but also medicine, reinforcing the age-old belief that good health begins in the kitchen.

As we sprinkle the final pinch of wisdom into this flavorful exploration of **10 medicinal spices in every Indian kitchen**, it's time to marvel at the true magic of these everyday ingredients. Turmeric's golden glow, ginger's fiery zest, cumin's earthy comfort, and the bold kick of black pepper—each spice is a tiny powerhouse, brimming with ancient secrets and modern benefits. They've been silently elevating our meals while quietly healing our bodies for centuries, proving that good health isn't always found in prescriptions but in traditions.

This journey through the spice rack is more than a culinary adventure—it's a celebration of how simple, natural remedies can transform our lives. Whether you're brewing a soothing clove tea for a cold, blending coriander leaves into a detox juice, or massaging aching joints with cumin oil, these spices offer a universe of healing possibilities.

So, next time you reach for that jar of cinnamon or a handful of fennel, pause for a moment to appreciate the power packed within. Your kitchen isn't just a cooking space—it's a pharmacy, a sanctuary, and a doorway to a healthier you. Go ahead, stir in the spices of tradition, and let their magic enrich your mind, body, and soul

Scientific References

Turmeric (Curcuma longa)

1. Aggarwal, B. B., & Sung, B. (2009). *Pharmacological basis for the role of curcumin in chronic diseases: An age-old spice with modern targets.* Trends in Pharmacological Sciences, 30(2), 85-94. https://doi.org/10.1016/j.tips.2008.11.002

2. Hewlings, S. J., & Kalman, D. S. (2017). *Curcumin: A review of its effects on human health.* Foods, 6(10), 92. https://doi.org/10.3390/foods6100092

3. Prasad, S., Gupta, S. C., Tyagi, A. K., & Aggarwal, B. B. (2014). *Curcumin, a component of golden spice: From bedside to bench and back.* Biotechnology Advances, 32(6), 1053-1064. https://doi.org/10.1016/j.biotechadv.2014.04.004

Ginger (Zingiber officinale)

4. Mao, Q. Q., Xu, X. Y., Cao, S. Y., Gan, R. Y., Corke, H., Beta, T., & Li, H. B. (2019). *Bioactive compounds and bioactivities of ginger (Zingiber officinale Roscoe).* Foods, 8(6), 185. https://doi.org/10.3390/foods8060185

5. Bode, A. M., & Dong, Z. (2011). *The amazing and mighty ginger.* Herbal Medicine: Biomolecular and Clinical Aspects (2nd ed.). CRC Press.

6. Lete, I., & Allué, J. (2016). *The effectiveness of ginger in the prevention of nausea and vomiting during pregnancy and*

chemotherapy. Integrative Medicine Insights, 11, 11-17. https://doi.org/10.4137/IMI.S36273

Cumin (Cuminum cyminum)

7. Srinivasan, K. (2018). *Cumin (Cuminum cyminum) and its beneficial health effects: A review.* Food Research International, 113, 153-161. https://doi.org/10.1016/j.foodres.2018.07.041

8. Panwar, R., Sharma, S., & Joshi, S. C. (2015). *Protective role of cumin (Cuminum cyminum) against gastric toxicity of aspirin in male albino rats.* Toxicology International, 22(2), 152-157. https://doi.org/10.4103/0971-6580.172257

Coriander (Coriandrum sativum)

9. Sahib, N. G., Saari, N., Ismail, A., Khatib, A., Mahomoodally, F. M., & Abdul Hamid, A. (2013). *Plants' metabolites as potential anti-obesity agents.* The Scientific World Journal, 2013, 436462. https://doi.org/10.1155/2013/436462

10. Wangensteen, H., Samuelsen, A. B., & Malterud, K. E. (2004). *Antioxidant activity in extracts from coriander.* Food Chemistry, 88(2), 293-297. https://doi.org/10.1016/j.foodchem.2004.01.047

Fenugreek (Trigonella foenum-graecum)

11. Neelakantan, N., Narayanan, M., de Souza, R. J., & van Dam, R. M. (2014). *Effect of fenugreek (Trigonella foenum-graecum L.) intake on glycemia: A meta-analysis of*

clinical trials. Nutrition Journal, 13(1), 7. https://doi.org/10.1186/1475-2891-13-7

12. Basch, E., Ulbricht, C., Kuo, G., Szapary, P., & Smith, M. (2003). *Therapeutic applications of fenugreek.* Alternative Medicine Review, 8(1), 20-27.

Cinnamon (Cinnamomum verum)

13. Ranasinghe, P., Jayawardana, R., Galappatthy, P., Katulanda, P., & Constantine, G. R. (2012). *Efficacy and safety of 'true' cinnamon (Cinnamomum zeylanicum) as a lipid-lowering agent: A systematic review and meta-analysis.* BMC Complementary and Alternative Medicine, 12(1), 137. https://doi.org/10.1186/1472-6882-12-137

14. Kirkham, S., Akilen, R., Sharma, S., & Tsiami, A. (2009). *The potential of cinnamon to reduce blood glucose levels in patients with type 2 diabetes and insulin resistance.* Diabetes, Obesity and Metabolism, 11(12), 1100-1113. https://doi.org/10.1111/j.1463-1326.2009.01094.x

Cloves (Syzygium aromaticum)

15. Chaieb, K., Hajlaoui, H., Zmantar, T., Kahla-Nakbi, A. B., Rouabhia, M., Mahdouani, K., & Bakhrouf, A. (2007). *The chemical composition and biological activity of clove essential oil, Eugenia caryophyllata (Syzigium aromaticum L. Myrtaceae): A short review.* Phytotherapy Research, 21(6), 501-506. https://doi.org/10.1002/ptr.2124

16. Kumar, G., Karthik, L., & Rao, K. V. B. (2010). *Antimicrobial activity of Syzygium aromaticum (clove) against*

bacterial pathogens of periodontitis. International Journal of Pharma and Bio Sciences, 1(2), B1-B7.

Black Pepper (Piper nigrum)

17. Vijayakumar, R. S., Surya, D., & Nalini, N. (2004). *Antioxidant efficacy of black pepper (Piper nigrum L.) and piperine in rats with high-fat diet-induced oxidative stress.* Redox Report, 9(2), 105-110. https://doi.org/10.1179/135100004225003897

18. Srinivasan, K. (2007). *Black pepper and its pungent principle-piperine: A review of diverse physiological effects.* Critical Reviews in Food Science and Nutrition, 47(8), 735-748. https://doi.org/10.1080/10408390601062054

Cardamom (Elettaria cardamomum)

19. Verma, S. K., Jain, V., & Katewa, S. S. (2009). *Blood pressure lowering, fibrinolysis enhancing and antioxidant activities of cardamom (Elettaria cardamomum).* Indian Journal of Biochemistry & Biophysics, 46(6), 503-506.

20. Jamal, J. A., Houghton, P. J., Milligan, S. R., & Ibrahim, J. (2006). *Cardamom extract as a potential inhibitor of human platelet aggregation.* Journal of Ethnopharmacology, 105(1-2), 219-223. https://doi.org/10.1016/j.jep.2005.10.017

Books on Ayurveda and Medicinal Spices

1. Dash, Vaidya Bhagwan, *Ayurvedic Materia Medica: A Comprehensive Guide to Ayurvedic Herbal Medicine,* Concept Publishing, 1991.

2. Lad, Vasant, *The Complete Book of Ayurvedic Home Remedies*, Three Rivers Press, 1998.

3. Pole, Sebastian, *Ayurvedic Medicine: The Principles of Traditional Practice*, Singing Dragon, 2013.

4. Sharma, P.V., *Dravyaguna Vijnana* (Volumes 1 & 2), Chaukhambha Publications, 2001.

5. Tirtha, Swami Sadashiva, *The Ayurveda Encyclopedia: Natural Secrets to Healing, Prevention, & Longevity*, Ayurveda Holistic Center Press, 2007.

6. Groves, Marlowe, *Healing Spices: How to Use 50 Everyday and Exotic Spices to Boost Health and Beat Disease*, Little, Brown Spark, 2011.